FEEL AWESOME
EVERYDAY

A Fun Guide to Basic Health and Wellness and
Living Your Happiest, Healthiest, Fullest Life from
a bartender turned Chinese Medicine Doctor

Dr. Sarah Pigeon, DACM, LAc

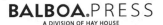

BALBOA.PRESS
A DIVISION OF HAY HOUSE

Balboa Press books may be ordered through booksellers or by contacting:

Balboa Press
A Division of Hay House
1663 Liberty Drive
Bloomington, IN 47403
www.balboapress.com
844-682-1282

Because of the dynamic nature of the Internet, any web addresses or links contained in this book may have changed since publication and may no longer be valid. The views expressed in this work are solely those of the author and do not necessarily reflect the views of the publisher, and the publisher hereby disclaims any responsibility for them.

The author of this book does not dispense medical advice or prescribe the use of any technique as a form of treatment for physical, emotional, or medical problems without the advice of a physician, either directly or indirectly. The intent of the author is only to offer information of a general nature to help you in your quest for emotional and spiritual well-being. In the event you use any of the information in this book for yourself, which is your constitutional right, the author and the publisher assume no responsibility for your actions.

Any people depicted in stock imagery provided by Getty Images are models, and such images are being used for illustrative purposes only.
Certain stock imagery © Getty Images.

Front cover image by: Jenna Benetiz of ANZA foto & film

Print information available on the last page.

ISBN: 978-1-9822-6364-5 (sc)
ISBN: 978-1-9822-6365-2 (e)

Balboa Press rev. date: 02/24/2021

INTRODUCTION

I WROTE THIS BECAUSE I LOVE helping people feel better. I love feeling great and it makes me so happy to help someone else feel even just a little better. That's why I do what I do and that's why I wrote this book. The more people I can reach, the better. This is a guide to help you live the happiest, healthiest, fullest life possible. I am always here to help and this is simply a compilation of lessons I've learned throughout my life and what has helped people I know live their lives to the fullest. My mission is to help as many people as I can attain optimal health and well being, so here are some tips on how to do that.

You know when you have the flu or are sick and when it's starting to pass, and you get a glimpse of feeling better (even just a tiny bit) and you are so thankful that you're starting to feel better? You know it's not going to last forever and you're just grateful that it's almost over? I love that feeling. I don't love being sick, but I love starting to feel better. Sometimes we don't even know we're feeling bad until we start feeling better, you know? These things we've been dealing with just become the norm and we go through our lives not sleeping well or being constantly fatigued or with slight back pain. Then we finally fix it and all of a sudden, we're like "Wow! I didn't even know I could feel this good!" These feelings are what this book is all about.

So much goes into how we feel on any given day. It could be the weather, how much sleep we got the night before, the traffic on the way to work, what we ate, what kind and how much exercise we've done and even the change of season. If we can figure out a few ways to help us feel better each day, we'll continuously feel better and better and eventually *BE* better. Working with what's going on in our lives, the elements, and nature, rather than against everything going on around us is a good start.

Part 1

PHYSICAL STUFF

Chapter 1

FITNESS RECOMMENDATIONS

LET'S TALK ABOUT EXERCISE A little. Do you love to exercise? Or does it make you kind of want to punch yourself in the face a little just thinking about getting off the couch to walk the dog down to the end of the block? Well, even if you're the latter type of person, I'm positive you can find an exercise that works for you. Do you love being outside? Or are you more of a "watching TV on the treadmill in air conditioning" kind of person? Do you absolutely abhor the idea of running? A LOT of people do, so that's okay, but it is usually a good way to start, test the waters and see how you like it. Start out slowly with just walking and then try running a block or so. Some crazy people (myself included) actually enjoy running, although I wouldn't say I actually *enjoy* running, so much as I enjoy finishing a run. But if that's not you, that's okay. There are a million and one different ways to exercise, so let's move on. Maybe you have some built up anger inside and would enjoy punching or kicking a bag every now and then. Or, if you're like me, you love hip hop music. Maybe you'd enjoy a hip hop dance class or just want to lift weights while listening to gangster rap in your earbuds. Or possibly, you simply need to zen out and would prefer a yoga or tai chi class. My point is there are so many different options when it comes to exercise, so you just have to think about what it is that makes your heart sing. If thinking about exercise doesn't immediately make your heart sing, that's okay too. You will get there because you'll find something you like and you'll start loving it. If you want to get out into nature, go for a hike or a run or bike ride outside. If you need more structure or motivation because you know you won't push it as hard unless you have someone telling you what to do, try a new class. There are lots and lots of different kinds of gyms and most of them do a free or discounted first week or class. I would suggest going around to several to see which is the best fit for you. Getting out of your comfort zone is tough at first, but the first (and arguably hardest) step is driving there. Once you're there, you're in and you'll do the class, right? So just get there, and by the time you know it, the class will be over. Furthermore, the more you go, the better you're going to feel and then it'll become a habit and it won't seem like the most unattainable thing to do anymore. So here's my suggestion, commit to going for two full weeks. If you can do that, you will start forming a new habit and, as I said, you'll start feeling pretty great and actually start enjoying working out (which, I know sounds like the biggest lie ever).

Now, some of you reading this now are like "Yeah, I'm gonna do this!!! I can't wait to go buy myself some new kicks and some super hot new leggings and get out there!" And some of you are like "But I can't because I have kids, or a job, or my schedule won't allow it, or this or that, or whatever." And, some of you are thinking "This chick is on glue if she thinks I'm ever gonna start, let alone, enjoy exercising." But, most of you are somewhere in between. I find a lot of the time, people get really excited when they're in my office or sitting at the coffee shop reading the book thinking "Yes! These are all great ideas, and I'm going to get my life in order and start working out and eating healthy, and it's gonna be a whole new me," and they're all jazzed up until they get home and think "Wellllll I kinda wanna eat a cupcake and I kinda wanna watch *'Friends,'*" and then it's all out the window. But, I'm here to tell you, that where there's a will, there's a way. There are just as many excuses as there are exercises, so if you really want to do this, you will, and until you are ready, no one is going to make you do it. As I said before, you simply have to commit. Stop the excuses and just freaking do it. Find something that you're interested in and sign up for one class, or one 5k or one team sport. It's all about baby steps and commitment. Take it slow, but keep going. You'll get there, I know you will because I've seen it happen for soooooo many people.

When you're ready and when you want to do it *FOR YOURSELF*, you will. It's the same as when one of my patients asks me if acupuncture can help them quit smoking. My answer usually goes something like this "Well, yes, if you want to quit smoking. But do *YOU* want to quit smoking?" Seven times out of ten, they say "Well, my wife..." or "my boyfriend..." And then I have to say "Wait, I didn't ask about them. Frankly I don't really care about them. Do *YOU* want to quit? If *YOU* want to quit for *YOU*, yes, acupuncture can help you. But if you're doing it for someone else, you may as well just go buy another pack because most likely there isn't much that will honestly help you quit for good until you're ready to take the steps and make the change."

This same thing is true with most things in your life, including exercise and fitness. Do *YOU* want to make a change? Do *YOU* want to start exercising? Do *YOU* want to get healthy? Do *YOU* want to start feeling great? You can blame your kids for a lot of things in your life, and I'll let you slide on a lot of them because I don't have them and I honestly don't know how parents do it. I know parenting is one of the hardest things a person will ever do, but I will not let you blame your kids for being unhealthy. I also know you probably want to be healthy for your kids, if you have them. So it's just more motivation. However, I am also a very understanding and sympathetic person. So, I get it. We have school and work and kids and dinner and basically adulting, in general, to worry about and can't always make it to the gym for an hour and fifteen minute class, not to mention driving time and showering and everything else before and after. So here are a few other ideas.

1) Start small. If you have a crazy busy week and don't know when you're going to fit 3-6 workouts in, try to schedule one run (or class or whatever you want) over the weekend. Invite a friend or your significant other, or bring your dog. Pretend it is work and you have an awful outrageous boss that will get super angry if you miss it. Do that one run (or hike, or whatever) and then do it again next Saturday. Keep putting it in your calendar, as though it's unavoidable, a commitment that you CANNOT miss. Eventually you will make it so you do that activity every Saturday morning-as if it's as important as clocking into work, and after a few weeks or months, it's your new Saturday morning routine. Once you have done your usual Saturday morning activity for a

few weeks, see if you can add one more per week. Maybe Sunday? Maybe a day that you work from home and don't have to worry about showering immediately afterward? Look at your schedule and find just one more day. Do the same thing you did for your Saturdays and keep up with it for another few weeks. Keep doing that, as much as you can, and see how you do. Eventually, you'll fill your schedule with your workouts 3-7 days per week. It might take six months, it might take two years, who cares? Remember the tortoise-slow and steady wins the race. As long as you get there eventually, who cares* how long it takes? You're doing it for *YOU*, remember? No one else, so who cares how long it takes or whether you do one or seven workouts per week? Sometimes we put so much pressure on ourselves that if we don't have time to run thirty miles this week, why run at all? Trust me-I have BEEN THERE! I am definitely an all or nothing type person and it's pretty easy for me to just throw in the towel and sit on the couch if I don't have time to run a half marathon a day (that's an exaggeration, by the way). But don't let that mentality get into your head. Push through that and just do what you can, whatever you can fit into your schedule, whatever you have time and energy for, even if it's five or ten minutes today, and feel proud for doing that! It's a big step! Try it for a little while, then build up from there. One run on a Saturday morning can lead to another on Wednesday evening and then maybe another on Monday morning before work. By the end, you'll be pushing through 5+ days per week without even thinking about it.

*If you don't already know this, "Who cares?" is one of my favorite phrases. You will hear it again from me-many times, so just get used to it. But, if you really think about the phrase "Who cares?" it's sooooooo true! Who really gives a f***? Everything you do is done for you! You're the only one that matters in your life, so who really cares how you're doing something, where, what, when? If YOU care, make a change and THAT is what this whole dang book is about anyway! So who f***ing cares?

2) Accountability is key! Put it in the calendar or sign up for a class a few days before the class. If it is in your calendar as if it's as important as one of your many engagements, (remember your terrible boss docking your pay if you "clock in" late) you have a better chance of showing up. Furthermore, if you have to sign up prior to the class, most gyms will charge you a fee for cancelling or not showing up. If you're like me, I HATE losing money, so if there's money on the line, I'm going. It's a great way to keep yourself accountable. It doesn't work as well for your own scheduled workouts, it's more for if you're going to a gym or class. So, if you're the type of person that needs to be held accountable and you know this about yourself, start out by signing up for a class or gym time, rather than telling yourself you're going to run tomorrow. And always remember that "terrible boss" that's going to scream at you if you don't show up (use me if you want, I don't care).

Okay, I forget where I heard it (maybe it was an episode of South Park?), but one of my favorite made up words is accountabilibuddy. Get yourself an accountabilibuddy. I workout with my friends all the time, and if I feel like I'm going to let someone down, or simply miss out on some funny conversation, I'm so much more likely to go. Do you have a friend who also has a baby? Maybe schedule a walk or run in the stroller with them. Do you have a friend who goes to boxing classes every Wednesday? Tell them you want to join. You most likely are not going to let your friend down by flaking on them, are you? If so, maybe you should reevaluate your relationships-I'm kidding. But, plan to do something with your significant other, a coworker, a friend, a neighbor-whoever you think will hold you the most accountable so that you do not miss that appointment. And, the most powerful accountabilibuddy of all is probably a personal trainer. If you sign up for personal training sessions, they will not let you waste your time and money by not showing up. There are all kinds of trainers out there as well, you don't just have to lift weights with them anymore, so look into personal training sessions for whatever you want to learn or is interesting to you. It could be really fun!

3) Are you already a person who exercises regularly? If so, congratulations!!! You're doing awesome, and keep it up!!! But, if you're bored and looking to change it up, there are a few things you can do. You can try something new. Sometimes, that can be the hardest thing in the world. If you're used to cycling fifty miles a day, it will be pretty hard to even imagine running five. Those of you who are thinking "What the hell are these people talking about-biking fifty or running five miles-you're crazy!" Just take this section as inspiration to try something new later on. But if you're thinking, this kind of sounds like me-read on.

Now, just like anything else, everyone is different. There are some people reading this that go to the gym every day and lift weights every day and wouldn't dream of hopping on the treadmill. And there are some people who are like the person I described in the last paragraph that are total cardio nuts and have run multiple marathons, tris, ultras, etc., etc. So what I'll say for both types (and the others) is to get out of your comfort zone! Think about the hardest thing to you and then DO IT! If you think running on the treadmill is the hardest thing you can think of, try running on the treadmill for fifteen minutes. Then the next day do sixteen minutes, and the next seventeen, and so on and so on until you work yourself up to whatever your goal is. Always start small and build up, it'll seem a lot easier than immediately running for sixty minutes on the treadmill. If you've always been into cardio and want to start lifting weights, try a high intensity interval class that incorporates some cardio along with weights. It's a good way to keep yourself motivated if you think you will get bored or start small if you can't lift a ton of weight right now.

Remember the Coronavirus crisis of 2020? I'm sure we've all tried, but how could we forget? I'm also sure we all learned *A LOT* during this time, right? One of the many things I learned during this time was how to get excited about working out at home. For me, during this time, I totally got back into my running, as I had kind of let it go a little, exploring different kinds of workouts and gyms and stuff. But since they were all closed, I had no choice but to figure out how to workout at home and go for runs. On the days that I didn't feel like running, I'd do something at home. For a while I did my own workouts, lifting weights and doing burpees and stuff. But after a while, I got bored and uninspired, so I turned to the internet, more specifically YouTube. I had always wanted to try hip hop dancing, I just think it looks so fun. But, I'll be honest, I was always a little intimidated to actually go out and do a class. I knew I'd look like an idiot doing it and just never went, so I looked on YouTube for hip hop dance workouts. I figured, this is as good a time as any to try it out and see if it's something I actually liked and who cares how stupid I look in my own living room? I'm pretty sure my dog doesn't give a care whether I have the steps right or look like a bumbling idiot doing it. I was right, it was super fun, so I continued doing it a couple times a week, home alone, with my dog watching me from the couch. Then I figured, you know, if I had a baby right now, and I wanted to workout, I could possibly do this while the baby was sleeping. Or if you only have a little while and not enough time to actually drive to the gym and blah blah blah, try an at home workout. After the Covid-19 crisis, so many gyms started posting workouts online, so they have made it so much easier to find a ton of really good workouts that way. So, if there's something that you've always wanted to try, but are afraid of looking like an idiot doing it, or if you have a limited amount of time on your hands, do a YouTube search and see what comes up for you. I'm sure there's something on there that will spark your interest.

Now here's some other stuff. Are you injured? I have a lot of patients who come to me because of an injury. For someone who has run twenty marathons, to tear an ACL and hear their doctor say that they will never run again is devastating. Obviously, as an acupuncturist, it's my job to help them feel better, and I would never tell them to go out and run six miles. On the other hand, knowing how much I love to exercise and be active, I can't really tell someone to put in serious couch time either. So what do we do here? There are still many many exercises that you can do if you're injured. For instance, if you have bad knees, something that has low joint impact would be good for you. Perhaps swimming, biking, or the elliptical machine would be better for you. Swimming is a great option for many people with injuries. It is low impact, has no joint impact, and helps you stay relatively cool. It is also great cardio because it helps you regulate your breathing. Lots of gyms have pools now, so you can most likely find one in your area if you don't live somewhere that swimming outside is an option. If you don't know how to swim, there are water aerobics classes that are done in the shallow end so you don't have to worry about that. I frequently recommend water activities to many of my patients for all these reasons. Once again, we are all different, which also means our bodies respond differently to injuries and new activities. Make sure you find something that you like and always ask your healthcare practitioner for recommendations or specific movements that you can or cannot do while injured.

The main point here is to be active! If you're not already active, start. Start small, work up to more exercise, whatever you need to do. Starting small is much better for someone who is not already active, because you don't want to risk injury. If you're already active and working out, great!!! Keep it up, maybe change it up, if you're getting bored or burnt out, but keep going, no matter what, and keep moving!!!

Chapter 2

DIET RECOMMENDATIONS

*I*F YOU'RE ANYTHING LIKE ME, you have tried SO many different ways of eating in the past. I was vegan, vegetarian, I gave up dairy, I gave up gluten, I stopped eating red meat, I went pescatarian, I did paleo, Whole 30, no carbs, carb cycling, high protein, keto, and the list goes on. I got tested for food sensitivities which revealed sensitivities to almost everything in my typical diet and I gave up 97% of my diet. I've swallowed my weight in supplements. I've tried "treat days" and intermittent fasting. I mean, you name it, I've tried it. I've seen naturopaths, nutritionists, functional medicine doctors, personal trainers, and of course acupuncturists, who all told me to eat something different. I've tried all these different diets for several reasons. First, I wanted to see what would work best for me. I've never really felt bad in my life, but that doesn't mean that I could maybe feel better. I really just want to see how good I could feel because you never know. I feel great most of the time, but could I feel better than I do now? Maybe. I also do it because I want to know how to recommend certain diets to certain people. I basically want to be the proverbial guinea pig (even though I don't love that expression, those poor, sweet guinea pigs). But we're not all built the same, obviously. Everybody is different, which means every *BODY* is different as well. Some of us really thrive on a vegan diet, whereas, some of us may really need to eat beef and bone broth. I've always said you can be a really irresponsible/unhealthy vegan and you can be a really responsible/healthy meat eater as well and vice versa. You just have to find the diet that works for you, so look into benefits and pitfalls of each diet, to find one that could work for you. I'm going to give you a few points and tips about a few more popular diets to see which you might want to try. However, there are hundreds of different diets to

DR. SARAH PIGEON, DACM, LAC

choose from, so it's virtually impossible to go through all of them. You can learn a bit here, but it's best to ask your trusted healthcare provider to find a diet that is best for you. For instance, if you try one, and notice a significant decrease in energy, it's time to make another change, however, if you notice that you're sleeping better with a different diet-BINGO!!! Our diets have so much to do with how we're feeling, not only physically, but emotionally and mentally as well, so if you change your diet and start to notice small differences in how you're feeling (good or bad) look to see what the difference is and tweak it as you need to. Again, every *BODY* is different and many healthcare practitioners have a different take on what they think a person should be eating, so make sure to talk to your trusted healthcare provider and ask as many questions as you can think of. Sometimes we just need to get the thoughts flowing to get the answers we're searching for.

Now, here's a word on weight loss. Many of us are hyper focused on changing our diets for the sole purpose of losing weight. I have a lot of patients that come to me for weight loss and here's the thing with all weight loss goals, and what I tell them. When choosing how you're going to lose weight, it is extremely important to find a diet that is sustainable and that you will be able to follow for the rest of your life. It's not a "diet" in the sense that we used to know the word "diet" to mean. A diet is what you habitually eat everyday. This is a lifestyle change. You are changing your diet to become healthier. There are a million and one "diets," "challenges," "cleanses," "detox's," whatever you want to call them, they're basically the same idea. These will definitely help you lose weight, but the key is keeping it off. If this "challenge" isn't sustainable for the rest of your life, chances are, whatever weight you have lost on it, will eventually come back when you return to your old lifestyle and possibly more.

Furthermore, when you're thinking about where you want to be with your weight and body, know that it most likely will not work if you're depriving yourself. Depriving yourself of something you love is not sustainable for life. So, you have to decide, is the extra five pounds worth you never having a glass of wine at happy hour with your friends or eating spinach and chicken for the rest of your life (think Thanksgiving)? You absolutely can incorporate some "fun" into your life and also be very healthy. Most likely, with a few small changes, you can still release that extra five pounds and still go to happy hour occasionally. It's just finding how to do it in the right way (that means the healthy way) and at the right times. Once again, it's finding what's right for you.

So, here are some of the more popular diets with their basic ideas, so you can see if one of them may be right for you. As I said, it's always best to check with your trusted healthcare provider before switching any diet regimen.

1. Omnivore-Basically, you eat everything. Of course, this doesn't mean queso and cupcakes all day everyday. But, you eat any meat you'd like and whatever fruits, veggies and carbs you'd like as well. Why would someone choose this diet? This is the most common diet for Americans. A lot of people don't know how to do any other diet. This is most likely close to what you grew up eating if you grew up in America. Some people really thrive on this diet. Why? Maybe they weren't born with a super strong constitution and they need food to boost their blood and boost their qi (energy). In Chinese Medicine, eating meat is encouraged because meat is a great source of qi and blood and some people really need it. Others have a very high metabolism and need lots of calories throughout the day. Many athletes eat a lot of calories to sustain the amount of physical work they put in throughout the day and the typical "meat and potatoes" kind of diet is a great way to get a lot of calories (although I know plenty of Vegan athletes as well).

   Now, as I said before, you can be a really responsible meat eater, or a really unhealthy, irresponsible meat eater* and this is important because, not only does it matter for the environment and mother earth, but also for your body's cells and your natural health. So when thinking about which meat to eat, try to opt for free range, organic meats with the most natural diet and living situation available. Yes, this will usually be more expensive, but it's also worth it for your cells. Happy meat gives you happy cells inside, which in turn, makes you happier! :-) So, what kind of meat should you eat? If you're open to any and all kinds of meat, it's important to choose the right kind for you. Again, there is all kinds of information on which meat is best and which causes cancer and which causes high blood pressure, etc., etc., I could go on forever. But, personally, I think moderation and constantly switching it up is really key. Should you be eating beef and pork everyday because you've chosen the omnivore diet? No, you shouldn't. Even if this is the diet that is best for you, try to switch it up everyday, by incorporating chicken, fish, shellfish and vegetarian proteins into your diets as well. At least one day per week, have a "plant based" day and eat all plant based. You should always talk to your doctor or trusted health care practitioner (nutritionist, acupuncturist, naturopath, etc.) for more specifics and what is specific for YOU because I do not want to give any blanket statements. As I said before, every BODY is different, so I'm not going to contradict myself by giving advice for EVERYONE.

*This is important for any diet, not just the omnivore diet, so even if this specific diet does not apply to you, please apply this knowledge to your own diet.

2. Vegetarian-This diet takes out all meat, so you eat mostly plant based everyday. Within vegetarianism, there are many "sub categories," vegan, pescatarian, ovo/lacto-vegetarian, etc., so I'll talk about these as well.

Plain ol' regular vegetarianism means that you do not eat meat, but some eat eggs, some eat dairy, etc. Again, it's up to you. The benefits of this diet have been proven many many many times. Plant based diets have been shown to reduce rates of heart attack and stroke, as well as, smaller waist bands and BMI (body mass index). Why would one choose this diet? There are many reasons, in addition to the ones I've already stated for choosing this diet. Many choose vegetarianism for religious or ethical purposes. Personally, I went vegetarian when I was fourteen because I went to Ireland with my family and we stayed at several Bed and Breakfasts that all had cows in their pastures. As a child, I had never really been very close to cows, and once I did, honestly, they were just too cute for my fourteen year old heart to take. I looked in their big brown eyes and they just looked so sweet, that was it for me. I was done. So I stopped eating beef immediately and from there, I gave up pork and eventually all meat. I've gone back and forth, like I said, since then, but I've never gone back to eating beef or pork again. It's been so long for me now that I don't really see the point in going back.

There's also ovo/lacto vegetarian. This means that you eat eggs and dairy. The benefits of this diet are that it's a little easier, considering a lot of food in the US contains some sort of dairy. I realized this once I went vegan and started reading every ingredient label. I was very surprised to see that companies like to add whey, cheese, and butter to anything and everything they can. It definitely taught me to eat more whole foods because, frankly, it was easier. You don't need to read the label of an apple to know what's in it! The side lesson here is READ EVERY LABEL! Know what's in your food, if you're not eating whole foods (but try to eat mostly whole foods, please). Read any packaged label you buy, because you really have no idea what they're putting in there.

Okay, so that's the side lesson, back to ovo/lacto. Other benefits include eggs. I mean, it makes meeting your friends for brunch A LOT easier, right? I'm kidding (kind of, since there's always avocado toast). But there are numerous health benefits to eggs, as long as you're not eating a ridiculous amount of them daily. We were scared of the cholesterol many years ago, so egg whites are an option, but if you opt for yolks, there are lots of nutrients in them. Same with dairy, there are good things in dairy and it can be good for you. But, as with anything, the amount is really key. Too much is not good for you. It is also an inflammatory food, so it does cause inflammation. If you have allergies, the first thing they will tell you is give up dairy. And it's very true. We are all, as adults, a tiny bit lactose intolerant, so even if you aren't diagnosed as lactose intolerant, it could still be causing inflammation or making your other allergies worse. So, again, as always, as I've said over and over and over, moderation is key! If you are vegetarian and decide to eat eggs and dairy, make sure you do so in moderation. A great breakfast includes eggs, but it does not include six eggs, it includes one, two or three. Dairy can be a good source of protein and other nutrients, that doesn't mean you should be eating a wheel of Brie every night (as tempting as that might be)!

3. Vegan-I love veganism, and this is why. It can be so controversial and the controversy is so funny to me! Why does anyone care what anyone else (as long as they're not your loved one) eats? As I said before, you can be a healthy, responsible meat eater or vegan, or you can be a very unhealthy, irresponsible meat eater or vegan. Just because you're one, doesn't mean you're healthy or unhealthy. So, with veganism, you're eating all plant based and nothing that comes from an animal. So no dairy, no fish, no eggs, no honey. As I've said, I have tried all these diets before, including vegan. I was vegan for about five years. One major benefit of veganism is that studies have shown that plant based diets have lower rates of heart disease, which in this country is a major problem! Also, a lot of people have issues with the practices that go into animal farming and the environmental impact of it and how the animals are treated while living on the farms. Veganism is a great way to steer (pardon the pun) clear of that and decrease your carbon footprint. However, as with any diet, if this is your concern and your main motivation for going vegan, know that you will still need to look into where your food is coming from. Veganism can be challenging. It can be hard to find food, especially at first, that doesn't have any dairy or animal products in it, however, once you kind of get used to it, I have found that it gets way easier. Like most diets, the first month is usually the hardest. It can also be a challenge to get your daily protein intake at first, if that's something you're concerned about. Some of us need more protein than others, so it's best to find what works for you on a trial basis.

As I said, once you get used to it, it gets a lot easier. There are many really good vegan protein powders, as well as other natural sources of protein that you can incorporate into your vegan lifestyle and it can be very rewarding and have you feeling really great!

4. Pescatarian-Fish! Pescatarian is like vegetarian lite. This is where you are basically vegetarian, except you eat fish (and most eat eggs as well, although some don't-up to you). This is basically the diet I observe now. I have found that it works the best for me to be able to get the protein, energy and calories I need, as well as, be able to eat clean for the most part. Benefits of pescatarian also include reduced risk of heart disease, as well as, increased protein intake. So if you find (or is recommended to you) that you need more protein in your diet, you may want to try being a pescatarian for a little while and see how you feel. Once again, some of the downfalls of this diet are sustainability and the environment. There is all kinds of information on which kind of fish is best-farmed or wild, which companies use sustainable practices, where to buy your fish, etc. It can be overwhelming, but you can do your research. There are great websites like seafoodwatch.org and even apps that are helpful in finding restaurants and supermarkets in your area that carry sustainable fish. Once again, with this diet, I still recommend doing a plant based day or two throughout the week. I use fish kind of as a backup protein source, or when my body is craving it (which usually means I need a little protein).

5. Whole 30-Whole 30 tends to be a "challenge" for most people. It is designed to eat whole foods for thirty days. So basically, for one month, no added sugar, no alcohol, no grains, most legumes are off limits, no dairy, no preservatives, like MSG or carrageenan, no baked goods or junk food. It is not designed to be a complete way of life for most people, but to be done for at least thirty days. Most people do it this way, although it is a lifestyle for some people. There are benefits to it, including weight loss and clean eating, however as I mentioned before, since it is not designed to be done for life, it may not be sustainable for you for the rest of your life.

6. Keto-The ketogenic diet is designed to put your body into ketosis, which means you have high levels of ketones in your blood and essentially, makes you burn fat more quickly. This diet is characterized by high fat intake and very low carbohydrate intakes, or almost none. Depending on your specific diet, carbs consist of usually between five and thirty percent of your total calories. There are many benefits to the keto diet, and since it has gained so much popularity in the past several years, it has become a lot easier to do. You see keto stuff everywhere now. I've seen keto bread at Costco and there is an entire keto supermarket in San Diego. And that is all great, because the easier it is to get the food, the better the chance of sticking to it. However, the biggest problem with the keto diet is that some people don't do it correctly or do it without researching it at all. I remember when I was a bartender and people would come in and say they're doing keto and they'd order food and be like "Umm, can I get a burger, and can you add some avocado and bacon and cheese to my burger? And then, instead of the bun, can I get another burger? And instead of the fries, can I get another burger...with bacon?" That's not healthy!!! Okay, I'm definitely exaggerating, but seriously, not by too much. People who have not done their research, or are just opting to ignore the "rules" of this diet are in great danger of eating a very unhealthy diet. However, if you do it correctly, it can be much healthier than this terrifying example that I've shown.* *I should say, I did make that up, but honestly, I did not exaggerate by much. People would seriously order another burger in place of fries. I always thought, I mean, they know they can just sub a salad or vegetables for the french fries. I've offered both, but who am I to tell them what to eat? I'm not their doctor (but for some of them I was, so I definitely voiced my opinion to them).

If you do keto correctly, you will still be eating lots and lots of veggies, which is great! I ALWAYS advocate eating lots and lots of veggies, no matter which diet you decide to observe. However, much like Whole 30, keto might not be sustainable for you for the rest of your life. Maybe it is and that is great. But for me, and lots of other people, you will end up eating carbs at some point again, so that is something that you have to think about before choosing whether to go keto. Again, there are ways to have a "treat" every now and then, if this is something you're considering, and it makes it a little bit more sustainable this way.

7. Intermittent Fasting- Intermittent fasting has gained a lot of popularity in the last several years as well, so most likely you've heard of it. And, there are several ways to do intermittent fasting. Most (including myself) eat at certain times during the day, for instance, 6-8 hours during the day, so you're "fasting" for the other 16-18. For me, I eat my last meal around 6pm and then I don't eat my first meal until 10am, so my body is fasting for those fourteen hours. Some do fourteen hours, some sixteen, some twelve or eighteen. Once again, this is up to you and your healthcare practitioner. Other ways of intermittent fasting are to eat minimal calories for 1-3 days per week and then eat normally for the other 4-6. So basically, you would not eat or eat less than 500 calories for Monday and Wednesday, and then eat normally for the rest of the week. This works for some people. I know a lot of people who do it this way and they thrive on it. Personally, I love eating, so it doesn't work as well for me. I'd rather eat everyday than this. But again, that's me. Benefits of intermittent fasting include increased energy, weight loss and brain and digestive health, among others.

8. Carb Cycling-Carb cycling is kind of like intermittent fasting, only with carbs. And, as with intermittent fasting, there are a few different ways to do carb cycling. Some people eat all their carbs in the morning and then none at night. Others eat no carbs on Monday, Wednesday and Friday. As with all the others, it can be sustainable for some, and the benefits are quite similar to intermittent fasting. You could even try doing both! What?! Challenge!!!!

So, as I keep saying over and over (until you're sick of it), finding a diet that works for *YOU* is key. It's never going to work if it's not sustainable. A good question to ask yourself when trying new ways of eating is can I do this for the next thirty days? Thirty weeks? Thirty years? If the answer is "No," try something else. Ask your healthcare practitioner all the questions to find one that will work for you and try some new ones that you think might work. I'm sure you'll find one that works that helps you feel great and gives you the energy and sustenance that you need to thrive and live your best life.

Chapter 3

SLEEP

$\mathcal{H}$OW IMPORTANT IS SLEEP...REALLY? WELL, as it turns out, it actually is extremely important. The thing about sleep though, is that everyone is different. As I keep saying, every *BODY* is different so that means some people need more sleep than others. Also, as we get older and at different stages in our lives, we'll need more or less sleep than other times in life. The best advice I can give is to listen to your body, but we don't always know what our bodies are saying, so what we need to do is figure out how much works for us to get through the day without needing seven double espressos or feeling like you're going to fall asleep at any moment and crash your head into your desk. Ideally, you want to wake up feeling rested and not like you're dragging yourself out of bed every morning. I sometimes set an alarm, but I almost always wake up naturally about five minutes before it goes off. And on most days I don't set an alarm at all, which really is ideal. If you can wake up when your body tells you it wants to, that would be the best option. This is not accessible for everyone, I understand that, so if you do set an alarm, try to determine how many hours you need to feel the way I was describing, then make sure to go to bed when you need to to give yourself that much time in bed. When you wake up, you might not jump out of bed like your spring loaded, but you want to feel like you're awake and rested and happy with getting up after a minute or so.

The other question I get a lot is "When should I go to bed?" Once again, the answer depends on the person. We all live different lives and some of us sleep in later than others. Some of us are night owls. Some of us are morning glories. We work different schedules, we have different requirements and obligations. That's life. It'd be great if all of us could go to bed at 10pm and wake up at 6am, but again, not everyone needs eight hours, some of us need more, some need less. And, not everyone's schedule allows them to go to bed at 10pm. Some of us work different hours and some have to wake up at 4:30am. Some work graveyard shifts that don't allow them to go to bed until 8am. That's the world we live in. So basically you just need to figure out about how many hours you need to feel revived and go to bed about a half hour before that. I usually try to get about eight hours. That works for me. So I go to bed about eight and a half hours before I need to wake up. I read for a little while or listen to a meditation to fall asleep to help myself wind down. Like I said I don't usually set an alarm, I have that luxury, but I almost always wake up about eight and a half hours later and I feel great when I wake up. I've found this is what works for me. If I'm going through something or injured or sick, perhaps I need a little more, but again, these are things we figure out as we go along. If you don't already know how much sleep you need, focus on how you feel throughout the day. Do you have enough energy to fuel you through the day? Do you feel like you need a nap in the middle of the day? Do you get bursts of energy at night? Do you have trouble falling asleep or do you feel tired when you wake up? Do you absolutely *NEED* coffee or caffeine to help you wake up? These are questions to ask yourself to see how much sleep you need. If you're answering yes, you probably need a little more sleep. See if going to bed earlier helps. Start by getting into bed a half hour earlier for a few weeks and let yourself get acclimated to that. If you've been going to bed at midnight for twenty years, you're not going to fall asleep at 10pm too easily right away. Start slow, see how you feel and go from there. Give it a few weeks for each half hour until you have enough energy to get through the day and you wake up feeling rested and ready for the day.

I'm sure we've all heard of sleep hygiene as well. If you don't know what that is, it's basically what surrounds your sleep (both at night and in the morning) or your sleep habits. So, it's important to find what works for you to help yourself wind down. There have been many studies that have proven that looking at the blue screen of your phone, tv, computer or tablet inhibits sleep. So if you can, try to put the phone or tablet down (and stop TV) about an hour before bed and do something else to help yourself get tired. Insomnia is a huge issue in our society and we neglect sleep so much but it is so important. Lack of sleep has been linked to many issues like anxiety, weight gain, being more prone to injuries, and many others. Not to mention that it is extremely dangerous to drive if you're not all there. Plus, one of the main points I'm trying to get across is being present. And can you really be present when you're freaking exhausted? Trust me, it has been my experience that, no, you really cannot. Even if it had nothing to do with how you feel, the few things I just listed are enough to make me want to crawl into bed right now, so just imagine how different your life could be and how much better you could be feeling just from getting more sleep!!! Try making sleep a priority for yourself and see how different you feel after a month. Once again, like anything, we can always think of excuses as why we *can't* do something, or why it's not going to work for us when everyone else is able to do it. This is why I say *prioritize* sleep for a month. Put it at the top of your list and really commit to it and see how you feel. After a while, I think you'll see a difference and continue prioritizing sleep to continue feeling great.

If you're still experiencing insomnia (which I know many of you are) and these few things that I've discussed have not helped, talk to your healthcare practitioner about things like acupuncture, diet, supplements and herbs that could possibly help you sleep better. There are a million and one sleep aids out there, so make sure you find one that works for you and is natural with no or minimal side effects. It's not worth taking if you're just going to feel groggy and hungover or hurt yourself for it. There are many natural options that work just as well!

Chapter 4

KEEP A ROUTINE

$\mathcal{H}$UMANS ARE CREATURES OF HABIT. Our bodies thrive on routine. Your body likes you to eat pretty much the same eggs or oatmeal every morning at the same time. It likes you to go to bed at the same time every night and wake up at the same time every morning. I know that's not always feasible. We have schedules that differ. When I was bartending, there were nights I'd go to bed at 4am and nights I'd go to bed at 10pm. This is not ideal, but it does happen. If it's avoidable (as in, if you are staying up on Friday and Saturday until 2am just because you can), try to do just that. If it's not, your body will adapt, but it is still best to try to keep that routine as much as possible.

Okay, now I also understand that this whole time I've been preaching about getting out of your comfort zone and trying new things and all that great stuff. So, you're probably thinking (as I was when I heard this), "How am I supposed to keep a routine, but also get out of my comfort zone?" But yes, it is possible! I'm here to tell you that, yes, you can do both. You can start new routines. If you're not usually the type of person that wakes up at 6am to go workout, try it. Do it for a few weeks and start that new routine. You can also try new things in a way that keeps with your routine. If you always do the same classes (Monday is Spin, Tuesday Barre, Wednesday HIIT, Thursday run, Friday yoga), switch it up! Try the Friday Spin class or the Saturday Barre. Go to a different gym location than you usually do. Take a different route to work. Go to a different coffee shop than you normally do. Yes, you can get out of your comfort zone as well as keep a routine going. If you always eat breakfast at 9am, but it usually consists of a bagel with cream cheese and coffee, try eating a healthier breakfast, (maybe oatmeal and some fruit) at 9am. There are thousands of ways you can switch up your routine, while also keeping it a routine. Have fun in this way. Like I keep saying, get out of your comfort zone, try new things and make a new routine.

LIFESTYLE RECOMMENDATIONS

THE MAJORITY OF THIS BOOK from now on is basically lifestyle recommendations, so I've broken them up into a couple different sections for you. Feel free to skip around as much as you want if there is something that speaks to you immediately or read chronologically.

Part 2

MENTAL STUFF

Chapter 5

FEELING OVERWHELMED?

SOMETIMES IT FEELS LIKE THE world is crumbling down on you, right? You have a billion things to do and you're stuck at the office trying to send an email to someone you don't even want to talk to- "Ugh, get off my back. I saw the TPS report." (That's an Office Space reference, if you haven't seen it). It's hard. It's stressful. It's frustrating. How do you deal with all this crap? It's going to happen, it's inevitable. Of course, a lot of the time it depends on the situation and everything that you need to get done, but also the reason you're feeling overwhelmed. Is it because you feel like you have a billion things to do and no time to do it? Is it because your children are screaming and running around you and you don't know how to parent because this is the first time you've ever been a parent (which is totally understandable and happens to almost every parent, by the way)? Is it because you have health problems that you can't seem to get figured out or fixed, or maybe you've been avoiding the doctor altogether and are feeling overwhelmed wondering what it could be because, according to Dr. Google most likely, every symptom leads to cancer? Is it all of these or a combination? These are all wonderful and valid reasons to feel overwhelmed. But sometimes, we feel overwhelmed even when things are not really that bad (considering what they could be) when we take a step back and put things in perspective. But, your feelings are valid no matter how bad the problem really is, so even if it isn't something that maybe you'd regularly stress out about, it doesn't matter. You're feeling it now and that's all that matters. We can deal with it either way. How, you ask?

Here are some suggestions of what I do and you can try this. Not everything works for every problem or every person, so you can see which seems like a better solution for yourself and try it. If it's not the best solution, try one of the others.

When I'm feeling overwhelmed with a bunch of stuff I have to do (and maybe don't necessarily *WANT* to do) I make a list. I make twenty lists. I make lists within lists. I have lists in my phone, and on my computer. I have google docs and notes and reminders everywhere. I text people lists. I write lists and put them on my fridge. I put lists in the shower. I write lists for my fiance (ask him, he can't stand it). I write lists for both of us. Are the lists going to get your stuff done for you? No, obviously. But the lists will help you delegate which tasks need to be done immediately and which can wait. It is also helpful when you get to check something off the list. It gives you a tiny sense of accomplishment (depending on what the task actually was) every time you finish something else.

I'm also a huge fan of weekly planners. Not just the calendar on your phone (which is also awesome and I use that all the time too), but a physical planner. There's something about writing it down on paper that just makes it become more real. It puts it out into the universe that this is going to happen. So write it down in your weekly planner. Write down EVERYTHING. I write when I'm going to the gym (spoiler-it's everyday, except Sunday). Why do I need to write it down when I know it's going to happen everyday anyway? Because if it's down on paper, it sends me the message that it's just as important as any other appointment that I have, therefore, is going to happen because I'm going to make it happen. I write down all the emails I need to send. I write down when I'm going to the dry cleaner, and when I'm going to Target, then I write down what I'm taking to the dry cleaner and what I need to buy at Target. It also gives you a feeling of accomplishment when you get to check one thing off and cross it off the list, and that feeling of accomplishment empowers you to do more stuff. I've always said the more I do, the more I can do. It's a lot harder to get off the couch when you don't need to. Get off the couch now, and you'll see all that you actually can do once you start going. Once the wheels are in motion, it's much easier for them to keep turning.

Now, sometimes we feel overwhelmed, not by what we have to do, but just because of everything going on around us. Lists won't necessarily help in this situation, right? Or, can they??? Here's what I mean. Imagine my last example of what's causing your stress or feeling of being overwhelmed. You have some sort of symptoms and you can't quite figure out what's' going on in your body. Will a list help? Not really, but you can make a sort of "flow chart" to help get all your ideas and anxieties and worries out onto the paper. So think, "Okay, it could be this or this. If it's this, we can fix it like this. If it turns out to be this, we can take this action." Do you see where I'm going here? Once you get your "flow chart" out, you can see how you'll be able to take care of yourself and it'll help put things into perspective, that maybe it's not as bad as you had imagined in your head. Having a "plan" does help when feeling overwhelmed. Furthermore, maybe you've heard that journaling helps with stress. Or maybe you've been in a situation when someone told you to write someone a letter, but never send it, perhaps to deal with grief or a breakup or similar situation. This is along the same idea as writing it out. Writing out what's making you feel overwhelmed will help you to "get it out" so it's not stuck in your brain on a constant cycle of anxiety. Put it on the paper, see how you can help the situation and it will help you deal with the stress of it.

Another helpful tool is to try to focus on the positive. I know that seems like the easiest thing and the hardest thing to do at the same time. And I also know it's something that you've probably heard over and over and over again, maybe to the point that you're now thinking "I've heard this so many times, I want to punch a wall or something. So, how's that for positivity?" Trust me, I've been there. But seriously, I was talking to a friend the other day and she was saying how she always tries to focus on the positive (and I know her, she's a very positive person), but these few instances, when she got cut off driving, or someone was rude to her in a store, or someone yelling at someone else on the street, just stood out in her head and she couldn't think of anything else. What I told her was, you have to remember these things stand out in your head because they are extra-ordinary, right? Ninety percent of the time, and ninety percent of the people you come in contact with are nice, positive, good people and good experiences so that ends up becoming the ordinary. When you're staring up at the sky and you see there are a million stars, but the one that stands out to you is the shooting star, right? Why? Because it's the extraordinary one. It's the one that's moving, when all others remain still. The reason you can't get these things out of your mind is because they are the outliers. They become the extra-ordinary. Think of how sad your life would be if ninety percent of your experiences were negative ones and the positive ones were what stood out to you. You have to remember, it might seem like the majority of things in your life are negative, but I guarantee if you think about it, the majority of things in your life actually are positive, but you're focusing on what is extraordinary. When this happens, remind yourself of this. Remind yourself that nine times out of ten, you have had good experiences driving to the supermarket and you've had good experiences interacting with customer service representatives. Just because that one experience sticks out, does not mean that this is the way life is.

You can also apply this to your daily life and all things in it. Just because the faucet is leaking, doesn't mean it hasn't NOT leaked for the last seven years, right? It's all about shifting your focus.

Chapter 6

WORK LIFE

How to be a star at whatever it is you want to do.

OF THE 8,945 THINGS I'VE learned from yoga, one of the most important lessons I've learned is to do everything with integrity. If you're a plumber, plumb with everything you've got. If you're a lawyer, look at every contract with all you can. No matter what you are doing, do it to one hundred percent. Even if it's not where you want to be, if you do it to your fullest and give it everything you've got, I guarantee it will help you get where you want to go. There are all kinds of lessons you can learn from each and every job you have. I started bartending during my undergrad and continued through my masters and doctoral. I was a bartender for much longer than I care to disclose and I learned a ton of lessons from my bartending career. A lot of these lessons- time management, people skills, and multitasking are applicable in many areas of life, including my acupuncture practice and teaching my fitness classes and I am so grateful for everything I learned while I was bartending.

For one, time management; when you have seventeen people screaming drink orders at you, and you have to figure out where the chicken tenders are supposed to go, it's really easy to get flustered and backed up, and get nothing done in a timely manner. I learned that I could make a couple drinks while the Guinness was pouring, or that I could shake a margarita with my right hand and pour shots with my left and simultaneously take another order. Now, I use my multitasking and time management to get things done while I have patients. If I have a patient on the table, I'm still able to get some paperwork done in the twenty minutes that they're having their treatment. These might seem minimal or obvious, but it really does save time and once you start doing easy things like this, you'll learn new ways to save time and multitask as well.

How to read people, how to deal with unhappy people, and being able to have a conversation with just about anyone about just about anything are obviously applicable throughout life, but again, are all things I learned from my bartending career and of course are lessons I've continuously used throughout life. I knew bartending was not what I was meant to do for the rest of my life, but I also knew it was what I was meant to do while I was doing it and it absolutely got me to where I am now. And, I chose to take every lesson I possibly could from that time in my life, because I knew it was going to help me later in life. So just know that whatever you're doing, whether it's what you want to be doing or you want to do something else, is helping you on your path to get you where you want to be (if you're not already there) and look at every day as a new chance to learn more and absorb everything you can from where you are. When you look back on your life, you'll be able to thank yourself for taking these lessons and making you a better person now.

What am I gonna do with my life?

Ah, the eternal question-what am I gonna do for the rest of my life? Most people think they know the answer to this question as a kid. But then, as we grow up and things change we realize maybe we don't want to (or physically can't) be an astronaut or firefighter or dinosaur for the rest of our lives. A lot of people don't know the answer to this question if and when they start college. A lot of people don't know the answer to this question when they finish college. A lot of people don't know the answer to this question when they're established in their career. If you do, congratu-freaking-lations, because that is awesome and you have just made your life a heck of a lot easier for yourself. Wouldn't it be great if you knew from the time you were six that you were destined to do a certain thing in your life? And maybe you're one of the lucky people who does know that, but I'm pretty sure, if you surveyed 1,000 retirees, half of them might tell you they could've done something else and been perfectly happy and successful doing that other thing.

So how are we supposed to know what to do for the rest of our lives? Well, first of all, take the pressure off of that question because it doesn't have to be for the rest of your life. There are always more possibilities in life and new opportunities present themselves all the time. That's just how it works, so even if you think this is what you want to do for the rest of your days, you might decide in fifteen years that it's not the best decision for you anymore at which point you can maybe start looking for other options. For now, if you're trying to figure out what it is you want to do with your life, or are deciding whether you want to make a major career change, figure out what it is that brings you the most passion and put it to work. Yes, there are eight million books and quotes and memes out there saying this exact same thing. It sounds so easy, right? No, I know it's not that easy. Most of us are pretty multi faceted so sometimes it's really hard to zero in on exactly what it is that brings you the most joy, and is also something you can make a career out of, but with some soul searching and thinking and researching, it is definitely possible.

I started college when I was seventeen. Now that I'm in my thirties I know seventeen is pretty young and I didn't really know anything about the world just yet, but some of us think we know almost everything about it, so don't dare tell a seventeen year old that they don't know much about the world! So in my freshman year of undergrad, I think I changed my major about six times, maybe more, until finally someone said to me "Just major in Business because then you can do anything you want," which may or may not have been completely true. But I didn't know that, so I did. I changed my major yet again to Marketing and I'm glad I did. I had started bartending while getting my undergrad and after college, I continued bartending and wasn't really sure what I wanted to do. I knew a lot of things that I didn't want to do. I knew I didn't want to be in sales. I knew I didn't want to do something boring (whatever that means). I knew I didn't want to not make any money. But what did I want to do? I loved to travel, so I thought maybe I wanted to be a flight attendant, but considering I graduated in May of 2002 (which was nine months after 9.11) it was a little tougher than I had originally anticipated to get hired doing that. So I kept looking into other options and in the meantime, just kept bartending. I moved home with my parents and got a different bartending job. Then, I traveled a little bit and when I came home, went back to my bartending job. I'd look for "real" jobs (as they used to be called-which, to be completely honest, I can't stand!) in between. I'm just going to go off on a tangent quickly because people used to ask me while I was bartending when I was going to get a "real job." First of all, I'm sure they didn't mean it to be, but it comes off as quite condescending when you're sitting at a bar asking the bartender when they're going to get a "real job" as she hands you your beer. And second, I'm pretty sure any job is "real" if it makes "real" money that pays "real" bills, which we all know, bartending or any other job does. So I say, and it doesn't happen anymore, but if it does and you witness it, please tell the person to please stop calling certain jobs "real" jobs and acknowledge that all jobs are real. Thank you for listening to my TED talk.

Anyway, back to my point. So, most of the time, I'd work whatever job, that I thought might put me on a good career path, meanwhile keeping my bartending gig on the weekends, for about six months, and realize whatever it was that I was doing was not what I wanted to for the rest of my life. So, I'd quit that job and go back to bartending full time. This was pretty much my pattern until I was almost thirty, at which point I thought I needed to get my shit together and figure out what the heck I wanted to do with my life. So I started looking into other jobs and grad school programs. And you know what? Every job I saw posted on Monster or Careerbuilder or Craigslist, and every grad school program I thought about or saw on the university website, I thought to myself "I could do that," "I could be a librarian, I love going to the library and reading books," or "I could study Kinesiology. I love going to the gym and working out," or "I could work at the Humane Society. I love animals and I'm already volunteering there," and honestly, the list goes on. I mean, you name it, I could imagine myself doing it and loving it. And here's the thing-I probably would have loved doing some of those things because, as a human, I'm interested in so many different subjects and ideas, and most of us are like this as well. I'm no different than anyone else. So, knowing this, how the heck are we supposed to choose a career that we're meant to do for the next forty plus years? Well, for one thing, keep in mind that it doesn't have to be the next forty years. But, one of the reasons I chose Acupuncture and Chinese Medicine is because I thought I needed an absolute, one subject career choice, rather than my college choice of doing Business because I thought that having something broad would mean I'd end up bartending for another fifteen years, while furiously searching online and submitting resume after resume for museum curator and personal trainer positions (for none of which I was qualified, if I'm being honest). I needed an absolute. I needed something that I couldn't deviate from. I needed a "This is what I'm doing and I'm not doing anything else." However, once I started Chinese Medicine school, I realized that, even within this tiny niche of a career, there are hundreds of things I can do. I can teach, I can write books, I can treat patients, I can write articles, I can own and run my own clinic, I can be a mentor and offer lifestyle consulting, I can offer CEU courses, I can have side hustles like teaching fitness classes and selling skincare, all of which I do now so that I don't get burnt out.

The other thing I've found is that, as humans, as I said, we are all pretty multi faceted-some of us more than others. So this means we can get burnt out pretty easily. If your day is exactly the same Monday-Friday, you definitely have a chance of getting burnt out. So, in order to counteract this, try to explore different avenues of your interests or your career now. Are there some other things you can do that would fulfill you within your area of interest or expertise? Get creative, talk to other people in your field and see what other options there are for you. It may not be something that you're thinking of right away, but maybe once you put your feelers out, something will pop up, so just keep looking. And, in the meantime, if you're having trouble finding something that pertains to work or your industry, why not look into something else that sparks your interest? You can take a class at a local community college, download an app to learn a new language, or even take an online cooking class. Maybe it has nothing to do with your industry, or even the industry that you think you want to work toward, but you'll still be doing something that interests you and is new, so you'll be learning something. It's important to keep your brain and your body challenged and healthy. It will help prevent burn out and will still make yourself more marketable. You never know what your future holds and you may end up teaching online cooking classes yourself or opening a bakery or flower shop or something down the road. You don't know where you'll end up in the future, so just keep yourself busy so you don't become complacent while you're getting there.

On the other hand, though, you have to remember to be patient. Life is a marathon, not a sprint. This is something I have to remind myself all the time. In fact, I have a tattoo on my arm telling me to do so because that's how hard it is for me. I'm one of the most impatient people you'll ever know. And, I always want things to work out perfectly. I want the perfect life and the perfect job and the perfect home, although we all know perfection doesn't exist in life, so I've had to learn to let that go. Sometimes the Universe or whatever you believe in has a different plan than you do so you just have to go with the flow. The plan (and life) is fluid. If you're too strict and structured about what the future will look like for you, chances are you might not get there. It's like my fiance says, paralysis by analysis. If you keep trying to wrangle everything into perfection, you'll never allow yourself to get anywhere because you're too busy trying to perfect everything that you're doing. Allow yourself patience, mistakes and twists and turns to switch it up while still moving toward your dream. You'll get there, just allow yourself to do so, and don't stand in your own way.

Chapter 7

MOVING FORWARD

*W*HEN I FINISHED GRAD SCHOOL, I had a lot of time on my hands. I started surfing and going to the beach everyday again. I even took up golf. I was talking to my sister one day and she said "You're surfing, going to the beach and playing golf? What are you, retired?" And I laughed and said "You know, it kind of feels like it." I even took golf lessons and went to the driving range, and then one day, a couple of my girlfriends and I decided to go play an actual game. Now, understand, this was my first game of golf. Ever. It was a Tuesday late morning or something, so thankfully the course was not crowded because I was terrible. We kept having to let people play through because every hole was just taking me forever. My friends were much better than I was, but this was the first time I had actually played an actual game of golf. So here I was, swinging away, landing the ball in the trees, four feet in front of where we were standing, sometimes hitting a grounder straight through the fairway, but slowly, slowly (very slowly) moving closer and closer to the actual hole. I think I may have ended up possibly forty over par or something...on a nine hole game! I think we may have stopped keeping my score. That's how bad it was. The entire length of the game, after every time I would swing (if the ball even moved), my friend (God bless this sweet woman) would say "Okay, moving forward," as though it was a significant accomplishment that I hit the ball even five feet. We kept laughing the entire afternoon at how terrible I was at this game. It is just not my sport and it is definitely a sport that requires a lot of practice. But, how kind she was to be so encouraging to me and, of course, to wait for me throughout the game! And, what it taught me was that, no matter what the speed, as long as you're moving forward,

37

you're getting closer and closer to your goal, so don't stop. Who cares how long it takes? Let people play through if they need to! Who cares if someone else finishes before you do? I mean, let's not get crazy (or lazy), but as long as you're moving forward, you'll get there eventually, so just don't stop. You might lose momentum for a period of time. You might always go slowly. But whatever! Whatever you're trying to accomplish, just keep moving forward. Just don't stop. In the words of the amazing Dr. Martin Luther King, Jr. "If you can't fly, then run. If you can't run, then walk. If you can't walk, then crawl, but whatever you do you have to keep moving forward." Just keep going. I mean, you know how long it took me to write this book??? I'll be honest, probably way longer than it should have. But who cares? I finished, right? And now you're reading it! If I had finished it earlier, maybe it wouldn't have reached your hands, so there's a reason for everything.

If you're reading this book, chances are you want to move forward in life, right? Otherwise, why would you be reading it? It's clear you want to grow, make yourself better, make your life better, right? So, the question really is, how can you do this? But, if you knew the answer to that question, you probably wouldn't be reading this (and, chances are many other mindset manifestation and self help books, if you're anything like me). So for one, you must be ready to move on. It sounds easy, but you will have to make some changes to your old self. Now, I know this sounds easy. We're all like "Yeah, so long old me! Here comes this brand new queen (or king)!!! What's up, world?" I can assure you, it's not that easy. It's not necessarily hard, but it does take practice. It also takes time. And, it takes effort. But it is definitely doable. Maybe some pointers or ideas for this, you ask? Absolutely! That's why I'm here! For one, meditate of course-my answer for everything. Do some meditations where you imagine yourself in the past, how you were before; how you looked; how you felt; what you thought of yourself. How did you used to view yourself? Unhappy? Unfit? Not making any money? Worrying all the time? Doubting yourself? Fearful? Single? Lonely? Depressed? Anxious? Stressed? Broke? Unhappy with your body? In pain? Whatever it is that used to get you down on yourself, imagine yourself there, in that mess of wallowy sadness and imagine your new self stepping out of that old skin.

And now think, how do you want to change for the better? How do you want to see yourself in the future? How does the new you feel? Bright, brand new, shiny, happy, gorgeous, successful, confident, fit, happy, rich, not stressed, relaxed, pain free-however you want to feel, really sink into all these feelings and how the confidence and success and everything that you're envisioning makes you feel inside. Really fully dive into this new you. Look at yourself, look at how you look and how you feel in the new you. Then, look back on your old self and tell yourself "Thank you. Thank you for getting me here. Thank you for making me the person I am. Thank you for worrying for me all these days so that I no longer have to. Thank you for showing me how I felt and for making me understand that I don't want to feel this way anymore." And then, imagine yourself letting your old self go. Maybe give her or him a hug and a wave goodbye, tell them you'll always love them and that you'll always be thankful for them and for everything they have done for you. And then, as if they're your fairy godmother/father (which they kind of are) bid them adieu and fly off into the sunset as your new, successful brilliant you that you know you are and you know you can be and let yourself shine. But, you can't stop there! Every day, you will be tested. The next morning, after you have this amazing epiphany, you'll have to put on your jeans and look in the mirror. Are you going to look at yourself and wish that you were ten pounds lighter? No!!!!!!! You're not. That was the old you right? You're going to look at your beautiful self in the mirror and tell your old self "Thank you for taking all the self-loathing feelings from me. This is no longer my weight to bear," (pardon the pun) and then think to yourself "Damn, I look good in these jeans!" When you start to feel those old feeling creeping in, just acknowledge them and say "I don't feel like doing this anymore," and let it go. You will still have to go to the same job you had before, and you will be tested there because it is still the same job. The difference is that *YOU* are not the same person. If in your meditation you envisioned yourself as the head of the company, keep that momentum going! Don't stop just because you clocked in and went to the same cubicle you were before! That new you, the head of the company you, is still there, so keep up with that person. Keep that amazing attitude and keep envisioning yourself as that "new" you.

Now understand, from there, your "new you" attitude will constantly be tested, so be prepared to talk to yourself (both old and new) a lot in the next few months. No matter what you're trying to get the "new you" to recognize or accomplish, be sure to be gentle and patient with yourself the entire time. As long as you're moving forward, you're getting there.

Chapter 8

WORDS TO LIVE BY

*R*EMEMBER THAT ELEMENTARY SCHOOL SAYING "Sticks and stones may break my bones, but words will never hurt me?" Do you remember how old you were when you figured out that that statement was, in fact, false? Or when you figured out exactly how powerful words really were? When I'm teaching my spin classes, I frequently tell my students to focus on a word, any word, that's going to get them through this next interval. I don't care what the word is, maybe it's balance, or energy, or strength, or cookies, or coffee, or wine. I don't care, but I tell them to close their eyes, focus on that word, see it frontwards, backwards, in different colors, upside down, jumping around your head, moving up and down, and many others. I tell them to just keep focusing on that word and pretty soon, we'll be up this hill, I promise. One of my spin teachers (and friend) used to do this in her classes, so I kind of took it from her. I also heard about an Olympic athlete who focused on one word for each Olympics that she competed in, each time it was different and each time, it had a different meaning for her. Every time she trained, she had that word in mind. She had it embroidered on her bags and printed on her tank tops and sports bras. It was always a word that motivated her in some way, whether it was a reminder of a time she lost or an encouraging word or something that made her happy and excited. It was always something that pushed her and made her keep going...all the way to the Olympics.

My point with all of this is that words matter and focusing on a specific word or words keeps your motivation strong, whatever your motivation is. Keep focusing on the same words or phrases, be it, confidence, strength, success, love, fit, family, money, abundance, prosperity, happiness, and so on and so on; whatever it is that reminds you to keep striving toward your goal. This focus will help to keep you going. It's almost like a mini meditation to just keep pushing and just keep moving forward, one foot in front of the other, until you're there. You can choose words for different areas of your life. For instance, most of us are working on more than one aspect of our lives, right? So, for your work life, you could choose "belong" if you are lacking confidence or feeling the fraud syndrome. Side note, for those of you who don't know what fraud syndrome is. It's when you feel like you have no idea what you're doing and that you don't really belong in the position you're in and you're going to be found out any day that you're a fraud and someone is going to realize that you have no idea what you're doing. I have also experienced this many times. If you are experiencing this, tell yourself every day that you do "belong" in the position you hold. Or perhaps, you feel like you're well suited for the position you're in, but not well suited for the promotion that you really really want. Focus on the word "belong," and tell yourself every day that you belong in that position. You're good at what you do and you wouldn't be there if you weren't. You know more than you think you do and you know what you're doing, so tell yourself that, and believe it when you say it.

Maybe you're simultaneously working on your body as well. #fitlife anyone? For your body issues, focus on the word "strength." Everytime you work out, think about your body leaning out and toning up, focus on the muscle you are using. If you're running, focus on your legs thinning out, dropping weight and your muscles getting more and more defined. Focus on how strong your body is to even get you through the workout. Not everyone can do what you're doing, you're so strong! Every time you use a different muscle, think about that one specific muscle getting more toned and defined. Think about the "strength" within you pushing you to finish that extra mile, or do one more set of curls. Think about the "strength" within you getting you out of bed in the morning to make it to your workout, where you might want to stay in bed or to get you to the gym after a long hard day of work. Focus on your "strength" that keeps you going. Think how your delicious, healthy meals are making you stronger, nourishing your body and replenishing all the energy you just used or will be using in these workouts. It'll continue to get easier and easier and you will make it happen. Whatever you want to happen, you can and will make it happen because you're strong, you belong where you want to be and when you put out your desire into the universe, it ignites a flame to get you there. It may not happen tomorrow, it may not happen when you want it to, but it can and will happen as long as you stay motivated and stay focused on your motivating words, phrases and keep doing what you need to do to get yourself where you want to be!

Words are so powerful and how you talk to yourself makes a huge difference in how you feel on any given day. Be careful with the words you choose and treat yourself like you would your best friend. Would you tell your best friend that he or she is never going to find the love of their life or get married? Would you tell your best friend that he or she is ugly or doesn't look good today? Would you tell your best friend that he or she is stupid when they've made a mistake? All these terrible things we say to ourselves have a significant impact on how we are feeling and achieving our goals. Do you really think you'll ever get a promotion if you tell yourself you're too dumb and never going to get a promotion? Start talking to yourself like you would talk to your best friend. I know we've all been our best friend's cheerleader once in a while (if not always), so be your own cheerleader. Motivate yourself with your own words. Even if it doesn't actually help anything (which it will, I promise) at least you'll make yourself feel better, right?

Chapter 9

WRITE IT DOWN

$\mathcal{S}$OMETIMES WHEN I'M LYING IN bed at night my mind starts wandering. That happens a lot when you have a fiance that snores (and that's an entire other topic), but it also happened before he and I dated. In this time, when I'd be lying in bed awake at night, I'd visualize my future. And in these visualizations, I'd think about many things...I'd see my house, and our cars, and my dream vacations. I'd see our yard, and our dogs running around the yard and trips to places I've always wanted to visit. I'd visualize my office and my days there. I'd see my assistant and my patients and my clothes and the shoes that I was wearing to my office. Then I'd see myself doing all the things I've always wanted to do, and being successful and excited and happy. It doesn't sound like I sleep very well, but I actually do. And during all these visualizations I'd get these little images or specks of ideas of what my next step was, or small things I needed to do in order to build up to this dream life that I was concocting in my head. If these ideas didn't come to me during my fun visualization playtime, I'd really think about it later and think to myself, what do I need to do in order to get myself there, and I'd brainstorm ideas of how to start making enough money to buy my dream house or what I needed to do now in order to eventually open my own wellness center. So all I did for each of these ideas was write them down. I wrote down every idea that came to my head, whether it was something I needed to post on social media or an email I needed to write or something I needed to research. Whatever step I needed to take in order to make something else happen, I wrote it down.

When you write something down, it puts it out into the universe almost like a little vision board or prayer. I've already talked about vision boards and lists and those are great! Keep up with those always! What I mean here is simply ideas or small goals you want to accomplish. Do you have a crazy (or not so crazy at all) idea for something that you want to make come to fruition in the future? Write it down! Not only does it put it out into the Universe, but when you have no choice but to look at things that you have written, telling yourself to do something or reminding yourself to go somewhere or research something or whatever it is, you can't ignore it. This little note staring you in the face is like someone poking you, telling you to get off your butt and make it happen (much like your vision board). It also helps you to keep focused and not forget what you're trying to do. It's really easy to lose sight of exactly what we're trying to accomplish when we have a thousand Netflix shows to watch and happy hours to attend. These little reminders are just ways to keep yourself on track. Do you think Alexander Graham Bell immediately started working on his ideas as soon as they came into his head? I mean, he kind of did. But he wrote down what he was trying to accomplish first, and then he devised a plan (and I'm sure he wrote that down too) and then (as we all know) tried unsuccessfully many times until he finally figured out how to do what he was trying to do. So, put it on paper, put it out into the Universe and keep focused on your path and where you're headed. As I keep saying, you will get there, just don't give up!

Chapter 10

FEAR-THE REAL F WORD

I GREW UP IN VIRGINIA AND we had a beach house in Nag's Head, North Carolina where we used to go for a couple weeks in the summer and usually some other weekends here and there throughout the year. Then, I went to college in southern Virginia and moved to Virginia Beach after graduation and spent many days at the beach there. From Virginia Beach, I moved to San Diego and have lived here for the last sixteen years. So, basically, you can say I'm a beach girl. I love the beach and I absolutely love surfing. I've surfed on a few different continents in several countries and I go as much as I can here in San Diego. I didn't always surf, though. When we were younger, we used to boogie board (which if you haven't tried it, is one of the most fun activities you can ever do). Then my parents bought kayaks and we'd take them out into the ocean and paddle around. And, of course, I've always liked to splash around in the waves too, just hanging out or floating on a raft or whatever. To me, being in the ocean is one of the best feelings in the world. I love the salty water, the way you can move around in the water. I love snorkeling and seeing all the fish and seaweed and rocks in the water. I love sitting on my surfboard waiting for another set to role in rolling up and down over the smaller waves as they pass by. I love riding the waves on my board. Feeling the rush of the wave and the energy of the ocean propel me along the wave, closer to shore. I also love wiping out or just jumping off my board, or boat, or cliff, or whatever I can, plunging into the water, surrounding myself with that cool, fresh, salty, crisp sting all over my skin. The bottom line is that I love being in the ocean and I probably won't ever stop loving being in the ocean.

There is a constant that I've noticed when in the ocean (and a point to all this as well), as well as, a question that I get asked all the time when I tell people I surf and how much I love the ocean, which is "Aren't you scared of sharks?" My answer to this question (and part of my point) is "Well, no, I'm not afraid of sharks. But, you can freak yourself out about anything, so I've definitely been scared in the water." There have been about 8,756 times that I've been in the water, where I look down and see the shadow of my surfboard (or kayak or boogie board) and think it's Jaws coming to attack me. I am literally scared of my own shadow. Of course, after a second or two I realize it's only my board, and I'm fine, for the most part, but then the idea of that shark is still sort of stuck in the back of my mind. If I let myself freak out every time I look down and see a seven foot shadow that resembles a prehistoric predator, or think to myself, "What if something happened right now?" I would never get back into the water. Half the time I surf, I go by myself, so I don't always have a buddy to talk me out of this. If I let my fear get the best of me, I'd be agoraphobic. I'd never leave the house. And that is entirely possible. It happens all the time. I can freak myself out about anything really. If I'm just walking my dogs, I can freak myself out if I think about any serial killer I've ever heard of. If I thought about all the car accidents that happen on a daily basis, would I ever want to drive my car? Probably not. My point is, fear is always there, no matter what. There is always going to be something to be scared of and it's going to follow you wherever you go throughout your life, whatever you do, or whichever endeavor you choose to seek out if you let it. The difference is what you choose to do with this fear. It is your own fear, in your own head. You can think of all the different scenarios that *could* happen. Or all the things that *could* go wrong. And, you *could* let the fear of these scenarios paralyze you and stop you from ever trying anything new or ever taking a risk. But you also have the choice as to whether you're going to *LET* the fear paralyze or stop you. Furthermore, have you ever noticed how much people love giving their two cents? They love to share their opinion with you and they may project their own fears onto you, by saying "I'd never go surfing, I'm too scared of sharks," or "I'd never start my own business, I'm too scared of failing," or "I'd never try to be the next American Idol, I'm too scared my voice would crack." Does that mean that you're going to get attacked by a shark or that your business is going to fail or that your voice will crack in front of Simon Cowell? Maybe, but you're going to do it anyway, because you will never know how high you can fly, if you're too scared to take a leap. There's a saying that I heard a long time ago that goes something like "Courage is not having no fear at all. Courage is having the fear and doing it anyway." This has always stuck with me and I've repeated it over and over and over in my head when the fear sets in "Why are YOU writing a book? You're not a writer. No one will ever read it." "You're making skin care? Why? How? Do you even know what you're doing?" "Why are you posting this? People don't care what you have to say." These are all things I've said to myself yet I do this stuff anyway because I love what I do and I love helping people. The fear that I feel when I see my own shadow, or when I walk into the publisher's office with my book doesn't outweigh the joy and excitement and all the good feelings I feel when I'm doing the things I love or doing something that's going to bring me success or help someone feel better. This is why we do the things we love and this is why we continue to push forward and take risks to make ourselves and our lives better. Think about how great you feel when you do something that you love, whether it's surfing or snowboarding or finishing a marathon or getting a promotion, whatever it is, think about that wonderful feeling of accomplishment and that adrenalin rush. And, next time you feel that fear setting in, or someone tries to pull you down with their negativity, instead of thinking of all the things that *could* go wrong, think of all the stuff that *will* go right! What if you ride the most amazing wave you've ever caught? What if you start a business and it becomes a massive success? What if you do become the next American Idol (is that even a thing anymore?)? The point is, don't let the fear overtake you! Get out there! Don't be scared of your own shadow, like me! Do it anyway! Go for it because you got this!

Chapter 11

BE PROACTIVE

I'M NOT SURE HOW YOU feel about the word "proactive." For me, when I see or hear the word "proactive" I get like that emoji face that is half rolling their eyes and half throwing up. I'm not really sure why, but it kind of gives me slight anxiety and also a little nausea just hearing (or reading) the word. Also, having someone tell me to be proactive evokes quite a bit more of that anxiety and nausea. Being proactive is not many people's strong suit, I have found. Some people are very proactive and go out there and get all jazzed about seizing the day and making it happen, but most people would rather have things handed to them, than actually seek it out themselves. I told someone one time that I'm the type of person that really doesn't want to work for anything. I'm secretly really lazy. If I could just meditate my way to a million dollars or a successful business or a perfect body, that's what I'd prefer to do. I mean who wouldn't, right? Now, of course, I'm not saying don't meditate-I have an entire chapter dedicated to meditating. I would never tell anyone not to do that. But does it really seem realistic to meditate yourself to whatever goal if you're not willing to be proactive and work for it? As I said though, meditation is great and being proactive by taking what you can into your own hands and doing what you need to do before you actually need to do it, just to stay one step ahead of the game is also great! However, here's the main thing, the combination is really what is key. Just meditating will do a little and being proactive will probably do a little more. But if you meditate, meditate, meditate and never make yourself available or only open your store two hours a day, or commit to writing your book for two minutes a day or just imagine a job is going to magically appear in front of you without ever looking on career websites or sending out resumes or even inquiring within your company, well, maybe that'll happen…maybe. On the other side of the coin, if you begrudgingly do the bare minimum of what you need to do, just to get by, that's probably not going to do too much either. Imagine you just scribble out your resume on a piece of notebook paper and only pick up the phone when an employer calls you (rather than call them after an interview to keep up with them or send them a thank you card or check websites, etc). Or imagine you continuously call yourself fat, even though all you eat is grilled chicken and spinach and workout three hours a day everyday of your life. Do you really think you're going to get where you want to be if you only do the bare minimum and/or have a crappy attitude about it? I've said to numerous patients "You will never get skinny if you're always calling yourself fat." Like I said, the combination of the two is really what is key. Have an amazing attitude and meditate, while also being proactive and doing what you need to do is really what is going to get you to where you want to be!

When I worked at a bar in downtown San Diego, we used to have this one regular guy who'd come in four or five times a week. We all got to know him pretty well, he was really funny. He used to love to play this game called "Would you rather." Have you ever played this game? It's a terrible game. Someone asks you would you rather do this horrible thing or this horrible thing and you have to answer. It's usually pretty gross, but for an example, would you rather get attacked by a shark or a crocodile? And you have to answer this terrible, terrible question. I never liked this game (no one really did), but for some reason, anytime this guy came into the bar we *had* to play it. So here's a not so terrible "would you rather" for you to ponder. Would you rather take a chance on having something possibly happen or would you rather go out and make it happen, so that your plan is fail safe? Here's the thing, you can go out and do whatever you want. If you want to get in shape, you can completely change your diet and exercise everyday until you almost pass out, but if you have a terrible attitude about it the whole time, you probably won't see the exact results you're looking for. Conversely, you can have the best attitude in the world and just keep thinking to yourself that the universe is going to send you a job making a million dollars and keep thinking it and keep thinking it. But the reality is, unless you win the lottery, that's most likely not going to happen in that way either. You may get into shape, and you may get a new job. But the combination of changing your attitude *AND* going out and making it happen is really what is best. At first, this was a hard pill for me to swallow. I didn't want to do any of it. When I graduated from grad school, I imagined I'd pass my licensure exam, get my license, have some business cards made up and boom! I'd have a thriving acupuncture practice and people would be knocking down my door to come get a treatment. Was that the reality? Anyone who has started a business of any kind really, knows this is not the case. Yes, I did meditations on prosperity and I imagined all the patients coming into my office and myself treating them. I imagined having a thriving business with full schedules each week. This was all great, and it definitely did help, but the reality was I still needed to do some marketing. How was anyone even going to know that I was open if I didn't go out and tell them. So I put up flyers, I put up ads, I left stacks of business cards wherever I could and a bunch of other stuff too, and eventually I had the thriving practice that I had been envisioning the whole time. Would I have gotten to where I am if I had the worst attitude on the planet? If I had been thinking the whole time that no one was ever going to walk through that door and that I'm a terrible acupuncturist and no one wants to get treated by me, would I have had as successful of a practice as I do now? Probably not. And, if I had just sat on the couch meditating, imagining people walking through the door, without ever putting myself out there, or doing any marketing, would they have actually walked through the door? Same answer. Like I keep saying, the combination is the key!

One thing that really helped me was pretending I had this wretchedly, awful, mean boss (who, in effect was actually myself) at my office. I'd tell myself I couldn't be late because she was going to be so angry. And all the tasks that I didn't want to do, I'd make myself do them so that this imaginary powerful, mean (yet gorgeous) woman wouldn't yell at me. Even the worst tasks that I really did not enjoy doing, I'd make myself do, keeping in mind the whole time, my horrible boss. When you're in business for yourself, it's really easy to let the things that you don't necessarily want to do slide because you're so excited about doing all the stuff you love. It's not necessarily a bad thing, we all have things we love to do and are really good at and we have the things that...well, not so much. But, we must be proactive even with the things we don't love doing in order to keep ourselves from getting complacent and keep getting out there and getting stuff done!

Most of us have heard of the Law of Attraction, right? Have you ever really looked at that word-attr*ACTION*? It's called the Law of Attr*ACTION* for a reason, right? Not the Law of Attr-inaction (or something like that). I've never actually looked it up, but I'm sure if you googled it or asked an English teacher to find the origins of the word, there is in fact a reason and all the prefixes and everything else, of course mean something, just like most words. But if you just look at the word, it says it right there- ACTION! Just like the movies, right? Even if the actual derivations of the word don't necessarily mean exactly what I'm saying, if *YOU* look at it, you can understand what I'm saying.

Yes, the law of attraction will help you when attracting what you want into your life. But you absolutely can make it happen as well, and we do this through ACTION! So, combine the two and have a great attitude, meanwhile being proactive and see how much you can accomplish!

Chapter 12

HOW TO DEAL WITH STRESS

SOMETIMES EVERYTHING STRESSES YOU OUT, right? When you're going through something, or you don't know how you're going to pay your rent or your boss is screaming at you constantly to get whatever it is she needs done immediately! It sucks, I know. But, stress is pretty much unavoidable for the good majority of us. Most of us don't live on an island with unlimited funds and chefs and drivers and staff that take care of everything for us. And, if you do, good on you-that's awesome! So, because stress is unavoidable, we have to figure out ways to deal with it. I'm sure we've all been in a yoga class when the teacher says "Bring yourself to your mat. Let everything from the day go and just focus on your practice," or something similar in a similar class or situation, yes? And it usually works... for the hour that you're in class, right? Or maybe just the first five minutes of class and then you start thinking "I need to email this person and call this company and stop at the supermarket. Do I need avocados? No, I still have one in the fridge... Wait, downward dog, yes, I'm here! I'm present!" Don't get me wrong, I'm not knocking yoga or any other form of stress relief by any means. I taught yoga for years and it has been a huge part of my life for many many years. Yoga and all exercise is a great way to deal with stress and we should all keep up with our practice and exercise regularly, as I've stated in the Fitness Recommendations portion and many other areas of this book. But we need to have other ways of dealing with stress, so that, if we can't get to a yoga class that day or something triggers us, we have some other things in our back pocket so we don't fly off the handle.

As I said, a great way to deal with stress is with exercise. This helps so you don't react like a tasmanian devil every time they run out of iced tea at your local corner store. In Chinese Medicine, when our qi, or energy, gets stagnated, or in other words, isn't moving for whatever reason, it causes all kinds of emotional issues, most commonly, irritability and worry or anxiety.

I volunteered at the humane society for several years and of course I loved every minute of it. So I explain it to my patients like this: imagine a dog that is locked in a kennel all day long without being able to run or play or chew. This is why dogs bark. This is why dogs become aggressive. This is why dogs chew the legs of your dining chairs. It's because they need to move that qi and get that energy out, and if they don't do it walking or running or playing, they're going to do it some other way (usually in a way that is not to our liking). And, the same is true for us. If we don't get out and move, like our dogs, we feel the same angst and stress that they do. We just let it out in a different way than chewing a sofa (hopefully). And, peoples' stress shows in different ways, as well. Some people get irritable, some get worried, some get heart palpitations, some get it all. So finding an exercise regimen that works for you is imperative to relieving some of this stress. The Fitness Recommendations portion of this book will help you find what works for you.

Beyond exercise, we can find some things that can help in the moment. We can't always make it to that yoga class and sometimes stuff happens outside of yoga that really stresses us out, so how do we deal with that sucky stuff? For one, breathe. Take a minute, excuse yourself from the situation if possible. If not, just focus on your breathing for one or two full minutes. Inhale slowly and exhale slowly. Bringing your focus to your breath has a way of slowing stuff down so you don't freak out too much.

Then there's the stuff that is stressing you out that is not really immediate but still somewhat acute, not necessarily ongoing stress. Maybe it's an unnerving situation at work that you're not sure what the outcome will be, or perhaps a family member or friend is not feeling well and you're not sure what's wrong. These are very worrisome situations and, as a human, it would be nearly impossible not to worry about the outcome. However, I've heard that worrying is just praying for something bad to happen and

I tend to believe that, although sometimes I understand it's not what you want to hear in that situation. It's really just projecting negative, worried energy out into the universe, so, in these situations, in which you have no control, ask yourself what you do have control over? Whatever you do have control over, take all actions you possibly can to make the outcome in your favor. Maybe give your family member all the healthy food and whatever else that could help them. Talk to your boss and see if they have any insight into the situation or make sure he or she knows what you'd prefer for your future there. Do whatever you can to try to turn the tables in your favor and then at least you can go to bed knowing that you've done everything you can to help the situation. There are eight hundred million things we don't have control over, so really why worry about them? What's out of your control will happen the way it's supposed to, but if you take as many steps as you can to make it happen the way you want, at least it will help you sleep at night and could sway the outcome in your favor.

Chapter 13

PUMP YOURSELF UP

$\mathcal{H}$AVE YOU EVER PLAYED A team sport or watched a documentary on a sports team and seen their pep talk before a game? Do you remember pep rallies from high school? That huge assembly before homecoming to get everyone excited for the homecoming game and subsequent dance that weekend. Now that we're adults and maybe not a high level competing athlete (although maybe you are and that's AMAZING!!!!), we don't have team captains to get us pumped up before our workday, so we must become our own team captain and get ourselves pumped. Do whatever you hafta do to get yourself fired up. In the morning, listen to some music, talk to yourself in the mirror, smile at yourself, do a dance or a cheer or sing a song, whatever you need to do to get yourself to feel the way you want to feel for the rest of the day. The aim is to continuously keep your vibration high. Do these little things throughout the day and then when you have the chance, focus on your self care to recharge yourself and keep that vibration nice and high.

I say this with caution, because typically it can cause more stress than not, but go to social media and follow all the motivational people and things you can think of. While you're there go ahead and unfollow all the people and pages that don't bring you joy or that stress you out or make you feel any negative feelings at all. The mindful, motivational pages have some really great inspirational memes, so follow all the wonderful, motivational people and hashtags you can think of. Think of all the successful speakers and self help authors you have heard of and follow all of them. Fill your social media pages with inspiration, motivation and good feelings instead of doom and gloom and things that make you sad, angry, or envious. We constantly have to protect ourselves from these energy suckers and things that bring our vibration down, especially when you're constantly giving yourself and your energy to other people; whether that means in your line of work or because you're a parent, friend, sibling, consumer, or just constantly there for other people, just make sure you're protecting yourself and your energy.

Some of us are in the healing arts industry, some of us are the person everyone turns to when they have a problem, and some of us heal others when we don't even know it. We give and give and give and what happens to our energy as we're giving and giving and giving is that it begins to drain physically, emotionally, mentally and spiritually. So we need to make sure we are always harnessing our energies and keeping our vibrations high. It's really hard to always give our energy and pump everyone else up, to be everyone else's cheerleader, right? At some point we have to focus on ourselves. And we can do this through our self care routine. You've heard that self care isn't selfish right? You've also heard that you can't take care of anyone else if you're not taking care of yourself, right? Self care is extremely important to keep yourself flying high like the star that you are! One way we can raise our vibration is through meditation. Meditation is a great way to keep your vibration high. I start everyday with a ten or twenty minute morning meditation after I exercise but before my day actually starts. It's always in the morning because it sets my day up in a positive way to keep my energy high and focused on allowance and healing before I start firing off emails and treating patients and talking to insurance companies, billers, editors, students, friends and the list goes on. You don't have to start with twenty minutes. Start with five minutes every morning. Honestly, sometimes I don't get twenty minutes, sometimes I get seven and that's still great. It is still very helpful to start your day off in the right direction.

Another way to protect your energy is exercise (are you recognizing a recurring theme throughout this book?). Activities, such as, yoga, tai chi, qi gong and nature walks all help to harness your energy and protect it. Nice, simple, low impact exercise really helps you restore some of your energy and get you back up to where you want to be. Bonus points for doing any of these outside and/or in nature to really raise your vibration! More high impact exercise (as we know) does use up your energy, but if you find yourself getting a little aggravated at pretty much everything around you, it might be time to go for a run or to a HIIT class. Whatever works for you!

Furthermore, find yourself a healer that you think will help you. I see an intuitive healer. I get massages. Obviously I get acupuncture. I see psychics, I have a life coach, I go on retreats, I do sound healings. You name it, I'll try it. I do all kinds of things to protect my energy and to make sure my vibration stays as high as possible. When I notice myself getting a little down or my muscles a little tense, I know it's time to make an appointment if I don't already have one. I always notice a difference in how I'm feeling after I've seen one of my energy healers. If you can't see all these healers yourself, as I said, you can always do stuff at home. Surround yourself in crystals, meditate, exercise, relax, self massage, read, do art, write or journal, get out in nature, whatever you need to do to keep that vibration as high as you can and recharge yourself.

Chapter 14

BE RELENTLESS, FEARLESS AND UNAPOLOGETIC

*T*HIS GOES ALONG WITH BEING proactive. When I was first starting out, I used to *haaaaaaaaaaate* posting on social media about my practice. I always thought to myself "What will people think?" "What will so-and-so think?" "Am I annoying people?" "I don't want to be too pushy or salesy or in your face." "Do people really care about acupuncture or what I have to say?" Here's the answer to all these questions: Who fucking cares? Please excuse my language, but honestly, who cares? We're all doing the best we can, and if you're trying to better yourself by building a business, or branding yourself, or making a name for yourself, or whatever you're trying to accomplish, who cares what other people think of it? Most people that follow you are your friends and support what you're doing, so you'll be surprised at the reaction you get. Honestly, when I started posting videos and stuff like that, the response I got really surprised me. People I didn't' even think cared (or cared about me, honestly), wrote back things that were so nice and supportive and it really helped me to keep making videos and posts.

Along the way, when you start getting bigger and realize your greatness, not everyone is going to be happy with everything you do. Most likely, the reason they're not happy about what you're doing is because they are not happy with their situation, or something in their lives, and they're just jealous or envious, so they will have to deal with their own issues separately (I mean, haters gonna hate, right?). So, you really can't worry about them anyway. And if they are happy with their current situation and they don't care about what you have to say, they'll either unfollow you or simply scroll past it, so again, who cares? You can't please everyone right? No, you can't. Who cares? I've heard numerous successful people say they knew they were getting big when they started pissing people off. People who troll the internet are doing so because anger inducing posts get the most response, so they're basically trying to do the same thing you are, (which is get noticed and get their message out there). But they're doing it in a much more negative way. So do we really need to care about what these people say or think? I don't think so. That goes for social media, but also for many other avenues of things you're going to do as you're making moves toward greatness.

What about for face to face marketing? I already said how much I used to *haaaaaaaaaaaate* posting on social media. Have I also mentioned how much I used to *haaaaaaaaaaaate* doing face to face marketing? Waaaaaaaayyyyyy more than posting on social media! At least with social media they're not right in front of your face, right? The thought of walking into a place with a stack of business cards, brochures and a smile on my face made me want to crawl into my own body, curl into a ball, and hideout in my own stomach or something. Like I've asked many times before, why can't I just meditate my way to a million dollars? Unfortunately, it usually just does not work that way. I used to make goals for myself-I'd go to so many businesses per week or make sure to put this many brochures down per week and things like that.

These are all great ideas for if you're trying to start or increase a business or brand yourself or something like that. But there are a million other goals that we can use this mentality for as well. Have you ever wanted to do a cleanse or change your diet or lifestyle or stop drinking for a period of time? But, when you think about the right time to do it, you think, "Well, I can't do that month because it's this person's birthday. And I can't do that month because I'm going on vacation." So we just end up never doing the cleanse or getting healthy. Once again, I'll use my patient who was on a long weight loss journey for my example. She had to become unapologetic about her food and drink choices. Anytime she went out with her friends, they'd ask her why she wasn't drinking. They'd try to get her to take shots or share an appetizer or pizza (she had a fun crew of friends). At first, she was a little embarrassed about her choices. She didn't want to tell anyone that she was trying to lose weight because she knew they would all ask why or tell her that she's beautiful and didn't need to lose weight. Now, that is not a bad thing. We weren't upset about her having great friends who think she's beautiful no matter what, but she didn't want their views to inhibit hers or to hinder her goals, so she thought it best at first to just leave it out when she was talking to them. So, instead of going into a long monologue about how she was trying to lose weight and get healthy, she decided to just be "unapologetic and relentless" about her choices- and by "unapologetic and relentless" I mean that she just didn't give an explanation about what she was drinking or eating. When someone would ask her why she wasn't drinking, she'd just say "I just don't feel like it," and move on or change the subject. No long explanation, because why? Who cares? No one really needs to know why you're doing what you're doing, right? It's completely up to you whether you want to share. Sometimes, if we share what we're doing and why, it can be helpful. Most of the time our friends are super supportive and helpful, which is why we choose them as friends in the first place. And eventually, my patient did end up sharing her journey with her friends and explained why she was doing what she was doing, and of course, they were super supportive and were happy to share a salad with her instead of a pizza. And honestly, everyone can benefit from fewer shots in a night, so they were happy to join her on her journey. This was really just at first while she was "unsure" about what she was doing. This is completely normal. Most of the time when we're embarking on a new journey or taking a risk or doing something new that we aren't sure what the outcome will be, we feel unsure, so this is where the relentless, fearless and unapologetic-ness needs to come in. Once you've committed to something, get that feeling of uncertainty out of there and focus on yourself being fearless. Do everything with the fervor of a lion walking through the forest because there is something to be said for just faking it til you're making it. We've all heard this before and if you tell yourself you're fearless and act unapologetic, eventually you will become just that and actually have the confidence of said lion. Just be "unapologetic." Who cares?

Chapter 15

THEME MUSIC

I HONESTLY DON'T REMEMBER WHERE I heard this before, but when I was in college I heard the idea to always have theme music for yourself and for significant times in your life. Once I heard this, I kind of committed it to memory and every time something else remarkable in my life happened, I was sure to commit to memory a few songs that will forever remind me of this time, and I continue to do this today. Whether it's a song that is playing when something happens, or it's just really popular at the time and you end up hearing it everywhere and it's one of those songs that you can't seem to get out of your head, you'll start to notice that every time you hear it, it reminds you of that time or event and then, there you go! You have your theme music for that time. Half the time it ends up being a song that I couldn't stand at first, but since it reminds me of a certain time, I end up loving it (think Justin Bieber, etc).

It's nice to have these memory triggers, but music will also help you get through certain stressful times and add to the emotions of happy times. And when the stressful time is over, it'll help you reflect and be grateful for how far you've come.

When I was in grad school, I used to listen to Ratatat radio to study. It was such nice study music because it doesn't have any words, so it doesn't distract you, but it still has a beat, so it doesn't put you to sleep. There were a few songs that really stood out to me, as some always do, even though the station can get a little repetitive after listening almost every day for four years. So when I finally graduated and finished studying for my licensure exam, I vowed to never listen to Ratatat radio ever again. I was done with that. But somehow, those songs end up sneaking back into your life. One day, I was in yoga and one of those songs that used to play on Ratatat radio came on. My friend, who I met in grad school was teaching, and I was practicing next to one of my previous teachers, who was now my friend and colleague. At first, when the song came on, I initially got slightly anxious. It brought me back to those study times when I'd question how I was going to be able to digest all this information and then be able to recall it later, and how many times I felt like that through the five years I was in school. But, as I sat in Child's pose, inhaling the sweet smell of my mat, I all of a sudden had this overwhelming feeling of gratitude and relief for so many things. I was grateful for where I started and where I am now and relieved and grateful for the fact that I was finished with the studying portion of my life and everything that had gotten me here. This feeling wasn't something I had really experienced before without being conscious of it, so as it swept over me, I just reflected on everything, and it felt amazing. This was all from a song that I hadn't really even noticed too much before. So sometimes, even without knowing you're doing it, you're creating playlists in your head from chapters in your life and when that chapter is over, you can be brought back instantly to it from hearing just a few notes. Be conscious of the songs you're putting on your playlist of life, but also, be open to adding new songs later in life, because you never really know when a song will come on that will remind you of a certain time. It may be a good time, it may be a sad time, but when you hear it, reflect on where you are and where you came from.

I also like to have different music genres for different activities, feelings and circumstances. There are songs that are great for road trips, songs that are great to run to, some that are on deck for sad times or stressful times, and music to just chill with.

For me, hip hop music checks most of those boxes. I have a shirt that says "But first, gangster rap." My friend got it for me, knowing how much I love gangster rap and hip hop. I always have. Anyone who knows me knows I love hip hop music and it has gotten me through several stressful times in my life. When I was buying my first house, I remember talking to one of my patients. I was saying how stressful it was for me-I was a single woman doing all of this by myself. It was my first house and I didn't know what the hell I was doing. They don't teach you this stuff in public school you know? So it was stressful, I was spending almost a half a million dollars that I didn't have, signing my life away on all these documents that I guess I'm supposed to be reading, but what the hell do any of them say? I don't know! My knowledge until this point in my life consisted of Chinese Medicine, yoga, dogs, running and cocktail ingredients, oh, and hip hop lyrics (and a few miscellaneous subjects here and there). So, needless to say I just had no clue when it came to anything Real Estate related. Going through this on your own, without a partner can be pretty scary. I had no one to turn to to ask what this means or to at least even say "At least we're in this together. At least if we're making the biggest mistake of our lives, we're signing this stuff together. Give me that pen." Well, actually, it's almost all done online now, so I guess it would be "Click that signature." Anyway, back to my story, I remember talking to one of my patients telling him how stressful it was. He and his wife were thinking about buying a house and I said, "Let's book you about ten sessions right now with me, because you're going to need them." And he turned to me and said "What do you do for stress? Everyone comes to you for their stress, what do you do?" And I said "Honestly, I run and I listen to gangster rap. I go through all my documents. I meet with my realtor and my mortgage agent and my heart starts beating out of my chest, and they tell me I might not get this house, this happened with my loan, we need to do this and this and this. And inside, I'm having a breakdown. Then I walk out of their office, I get in the car and blast gangster rap, the harder and louder, the better. And honestly, it makes me feel better. And then I go for a run with my dog." And he laughed, but he also understood. It's really always been my release. It relaxes me so much. I don't know how I would cope if it weren't for my hip hop music and it has definitely gotten me through many times in my life. So I will always be thankful for Jeezy radio for getting me through some tough times, including into escrow and subsequently into my first home.

Another reason I love hip hop music is because, when I first started doing all my self discovery work, trying to manifest my millions of dollars, I of course listened to hip hop music all the time. I ALWAYS listen to hip hop music. But this was when I realized why-why it has so much meaning for me, and why it relaxes me so much. It's because, if you listen to the lyrics, or even if you just think about so many rappers and hip hop artists, you learn where they came from. And I thought to myself, so many artists (not just hip hop, but this happens to be my choice) have come up from so little and have manifested such wondrous things for themselves. Remember how Jewel lived out of her van in San Diego? And Jay-Z grew up in the Marcy Projects in Brooklyn? All these people are so inspirational to me. A lot of people had so much less than a lot of others and have done so much with it and have made so much for themselves. It's absolutely incredible and such an inspiration. So I use this inspiration when I try new things or when I am about to take a risk. I channel my inner rapper, and I go out and do it. And that's why I wear that shirt, because, if I first listen to gangster rap, I get the motivation I need to do what I need to do.

So, much like me and my hip hop, find a type or genre of music that speaks to you-whatever it may be. Maybe you really like hip hop too, and if that's the case, maybe I'll run into you at a show sometime. But whichever genre speaks to you, discover as much of it as you can. Find some songs that really inspire and motivate you. Maybe you particularly like the beat or the lyrics or the artist. But whatever it is, dive deep into it and listen to it as much as you want. Figure out if you like different types of music for different activities. Most likely you'll want different music for when you're running than when you're trying to concentrate on work. Maybe not? But, just put on the music that inspires you, relaxes you, whatever it is that puts your soul at ease to accomplish whatever it is you're attempting and feel into the music to get done whatever you need to get done.

Part 3

SPIRITUAL STUFF

Chapter 16

PRACTICE GRATITUDE

$\mathcal{S}$OMETIMES WHEN I'M FEELING DISCOURAGED or having a rough day, I take a look at my phone and scroll through my pictures. All these great memories and wonderful people (and animals, and nature, and places) in my life make me feel so happy and I feel so blessed to have been able to have all these wonderful experiences. A scroll through my Facebook or Instagram photos will do the same thing. I like to take a look back and reflect on everything good (and sometimes not so good) that has happened and what I've been through and what I've done through the years. Since they're photos, almost all of them are good memories. But sometimes a photo that reminds me of a not so great time in my life pops up. Or maybe something that happened surrounding a certain event reminds me of a subsequent event or something else that wasn't the happiest time in my life. And then, of course, there were the times in my life when I was happy, but maybe it didn't end so well (I'm talking about break ups here, people). But even these not so great memories remind me of everything that has gotten me to where I am now and I can reflect on that and still feel grateful and truly blessed. After I go through my photos, or just randomly on occasion, I open a note in my phone and just start jotting down everything that makes me happy throughout the day, and periodically, I'll pull up the note and read it. Looking through it, I remember random things that brought me joy-a coffee that was outstanding and drinking it while walking on the boardwalk in San Diego; seeing a hummingbird outside my deck looking at my dog; the beautiful rose garden on my running route that smelled so good I always had to stop and walk so I could take nice long inhales and take in as much of the fragrance as I could.

One morning, I had just taught a Spin class at a gym where I don't usually teach. I was just substituting on a Saturday morning. Since I was subbing, I wasn't sure what to expect, but it turned out to be a particularly nice group of people (my spin students are generally very very nice and happy, this group was just a little extra). Several people came up to me after class to tell me how great a class it was and asked me to come back whenever the regular teacher wasn't there, and they were very talkative and interactive-just generally nice, happy people. So afterward, I was already in a great mood. The gym was near the beach, so when I finished teaching, I grabbed a coffee and walked down to the boardwalk where I just started noticing things around me. The waves, the salty air, the people walking, running, riding skateboards. I sat down for a second, and I looked over and there were two homeless gentlemen close by. One of them was in a wheelchair and couldn't see. The other was helping him eat and move about. The way they spoke to each other was so kind and, as people walked by, they dropped money into their jar. I watched this for a few minutes, and then, dropped a little money in the jar as well, and kept walking. It was so heartwarming to witness such kindness from so many people. The people walking by, willing to give them money, the one guy helping his friend and the other one, appreciative of his friend's help. I was grateful for so many things at that moment so I wrote them in my note so I could carry it on as long as possible.

I'm sure you've heard it before, but practicing gratitude can really help you reflect on how great things really are. It helps to put things in perspective when you think that you don't have a lot to be thankful for at the time. Practicing gratitude has also been shown to help reduce anxiety and increase happiness (practicing acts of kindness has also been shown to have these effects!).

So, if you're feeling a little blue, or just need a little pick me up-or even if you're feeling amazing and super happy, think about some things that you experienced during the day. Did you see a pretty flower that you loved or perhaps a person helping another person? Did you go for a walk in a beautiful park in nature or walk down to the beach to breathe the salt air? Or, did you eat a delicious piece of cake or fruit or something else that was just so good you can't stop thinking about it? Every morning when you wake up or every night before you go to bed, write down three to five things you can be grateful for or a few things that brought you joy that day or that you're excited for. Starting the day off with a feeling of gratitude helps set your attitude up for the day so you'll have this feeling throughout the day. In the same way, going to sleep having just thought about these awesome things, helps you go to sleep with the same feeling of joy and gratitude in your heart. It also helps to put your mind at ease before trying to sleep, so if you're prone to anxiety or insomnia, this can help with that. The fact that you're sitting here right now reading this book means that you have a lot you can be grateful for, it's really just a matter of tapping into it and switching your mindset to focus on your abundance and everything that's good in life, rather than your lack or all things negative. All it is is just switching the mentality from glass half empty to glass half full.

Chapter 17

EMBRACE EVERY MOMENT

I LIKE TO LOOK AT MY life like a book, or a movie. When I was a kid I used to ponder life in general (with all the wisdom I had accrued in five years) and wonder what if life was a movie? What if people were watching your every move and then when you die, the movie ends and everyone leaves the theater? I have no idea why I ever thought this. It's one of those weird things you think when you're a kid, I guess. But I guess it kind of stuck with me because now I still think every point in life as a chapter or new scene of life, so I look at different turning points as new beginnings or new chapters. When I moved to San Diego, it was the end of my Virginia chapter. When I quit bartending, it was the start of my acupuncture career chapter. I had my college chapter, and my traveling chapters. And I'll have my retired chapters and maybe even my grandkids chapter. I'm not sure what chapters lie ahead, but that's the beauty of life. If my life book was already written, my real life would be pretty darn boring and anticlimactic.

I remember when I was in my twenties "chapter" I used to worry a lot of the time about whether I'd ever find my soul mate and get married and have children. My friends and I talked about it a lot. We dated people and we asked each other whether the person we were dating could potentially be "the one." Some of us found our person. Some of us kept dating. It wasn't until I hit my thirties that I suddenly (and I'm not really sure why) stopped worrying about it so much. I had started grad school and I guess I just subconsciously realized maybe I didn't have time for it or something. Like I said, I'm not really sure why but we don't always have to know why certain things in life happen. Sure I'd have moments when I felt lonely and thought it'd be nice to have a boyfriend right now to go have some fro yo with. But for the most part I was pretty happy being single and doing things on my own. I was fine to go get fro yo by myself. No one judged what kind of fro yo I got (not that anyone does now, but still). I could mix peach sorbet with peanut butter fudge if I darn well pleased. I traveled by myself. I went out to eat and even went out for a drink after work by myself. It may sound sad, but it was actually really really nice. I really genuinely enjoyed being by myself. Even right now, I'm writing this book by myself at a coffee shop on my lunch break and loving it. I lived by myself and really, as long as I had my dog, Naya, I was happy. Eventually, though, I started thinking to myself "Okay, most likely I'm going to get married because a lot people do. But if I don't, I'm fine with that too because I determine my own happiness and I'm happy sitting on the couch with my dog watching tv drinking wine or eating fro yo solo. However, more likely than not, I will end up getting married and I know when I have kids running around the house, screaming and a husband sitting on the couch and snoring next to me in bed every night, I'm going to look back on my single days and think 'Remember how nice it was to sit on the couch in silence with my dog, watching whatever true crime story or Bravo show I wanted, drinking a glass of wine and later taking up the entire bed and having the covers all to myself?'" And I know when I have the kids and the husband, I'll be happy too. So I learned to embrace this "single" chapter of my life. And now I embrace all the new chapters of my life because I know every chapter is temporary and things are constantly changing. When I wasn't embracing my singledom I was yearning for a husband and babies and overlooking how amazing and freeing and fulfilling it is to be single. And now here I am with a soon to be husband, so now I embrace this chapter. My married (and engaged) chapter is equally amazing and fulfilling, just in a different way. So embrace every chapter. Know that the circumstances will most likely change eventually so see the good parts of it and enjoy them! And know when your next chapter begins, there will be some pretty awesome aspects of that one as well!

My fiance and I got engaged in April of 2019, and we were so excited, just as anyone would be. We planned our wedding for about a year after we got engaged, so when January 2020 rolled around we were REALLY excited- only a few more months! Being engaged was so fun. Everyone is always so excited for you and it reminds them of when they got engaged and they're just so happy. It's a great time in life for you as a couple. Every time we'd plan something else for the wedding, we'd get excited all over again and it was just so fun. So as February started approaching I kept thinking, I'm almost not engaged anymore. We're never going to be engaged again (hopefully haha), I'm almost going to miss it. Then (as we all remember) in March of 2020, the entire world came to a crashing halt with the spread of the CoronaVirus outbreak. Basically, the whole world was canceled for, what we thought would be, March and April and May, and that included our wedding. As devastating as that was for us, after I finally accepted that it wasn't happening on our original date, I had to think to myself "Well, I guess my engagement chapter isn't over yet. I get one more year to enjoy being engaged." So we did. And this time we really enjoyed it. We didn't have anything to plan, even though I really enjoyed planning our wedding. We didn't have to worry about money because we were granted a whole extra year to save. And, as I said, once we accepted what was happening (and really, the whole world went to crap, so our wedding seemed somewhat miniscule in the grand scheme of things), it actually started to feel like we had always planned on an April 2021 wedding. After April 18, 2020 passed, it felt like we had always been planning on April 2021. So it was fine. We thought we'd take our "honeymoon" before we were even married, but that got canceled as well. But in this time, we knew things could be so much worse, and we embraced having each other around everyday and doing things out of the ordinary. We couldn't really go out or do the stuff we normally do, so we took lots and lots of walks and hikes outside and talked about when we finally would be able to get married and how amazing it would be then. Even though 2020 sucked, right? No one is disputing that. We were still able to find joy in most things knowing that this time was given to us to spend together and get excited for what's to come and for when we're allowed to actually do stuff again. Don't get me wrong, there were days that I thought a lot of stuff kind of stunk, and I definitely wished for the days to go by more quickly so we could hurry up and be over this, but then I'd talk to myself again and understand that in this exact moment, things are pretty darn good and that's awesome.

Here's the other thing, though. We're always yearning for the next day. We're always looking forward to what's going to happen in the future; the trip we have planned, our graduation date, our wedding, Friday happy hour, whatever it is. I'm not saying don't look forward to things. Of course we have things to look forward to. That's the whole point of setting goals and planning. But my point is to enjoy where you are when you are there. I know we all hear all the time to be present, enjoy the moment, blah blah blah. So here's one more! I'm only semi joking, because, it is true, you want to embrace every moment because when you're in another chapter of your book or another scene of your movie called "Life," you'll look back on those other chapters and remember the good things that came from them and remember the happiness you were feeling. So you'll be embracing them as moments in the past, why not go ahead and embrace those times now?

Everything is temporary, right? So when it's good, enjoy it and when it's not, know that it'll pass. It'll all pass, whether it's good or bad and it's just another chapter in your book or scene in your movie, so know that eventually the page will turn or the scene will end, just make sure to take in as much as you can of this moment, right here, where you are right now.

Chapter 18

TRAVEL

*W*HEN I WAS WORKING AT a bar in downtown San Diego, the guys that I worked with gave me the nickname "Vacation Sarah." I loved that name, I mean, who wouldn't? They'd look at the schedule and see that I had requested off, yet again, and say "Oh Vacation Sarah, where's she going this time?" I'd come back and they'd say "Hey! How was Zimbabwe?" And I'd say "Umm, I was in Virginia," or "San Francisco," or something. They always assumed I was going somewhere super far away and awesome and sometimes they were right, but sometimes, I was just going to Vegas for a bachelorette party or something (which is also awesome). They called me that obviously, because I took a lot of vacations. I was in grad school, and my school did trimesters, which meant we had three semesters per year, with a two, three or four week break in between. So, I'd take a vacation at almost every break and I'd try to go somewhere I hadn't been, unless, of course, it was December and I'd go home to Virginia to see my family. And sometimes, toward the end of my grad school career, as I was getting closer to graduation, which meant I was getting more and more over school, I'd take another vacation even during the semester. I used to text my now fiance from wherever I was while he was in class and ask what I was missing and he'd text back and say "I'm supposed to tell you what we're doing right now, while I'm stuck in class and you're texting me pictures of the most beautiful place on the planet?!" He's very sarcastic. Anyway, I took a lot of vacations back then.

Most people who know me know I love to travel. I started traveling right after I graduated college, and I was bitten by the bug. It started with Europe, then I came back and saved to visit my sister who lives in Australia.

While there, we went to Indonesia and basically after that, it was all over for me. I got a taste and I never wanted to stop. I wanted to go everywhere and I still do. There are about a million and one reasons I love to travel. For one, it opens your eyes and mind to so many new things you had no idea existed. It is very easy to get caught up in your very own small world and going to new places, meeting new people and experiencing new ways of being expand your mind so much to see that there are so many other ways to think and live and be.

When I take another trip or go somewhere new, I always learn something. There are so many lessons we can learn from experiencing new things. I take these lessons home with me and try to apply them to my life here as much as I can. So, I want to share some of the things that I've learned from traveling:

THINGS AND STUFF DON'T REALLY MATTER

*D*ON'T GET ME WRONG. I do love my stuff. I love having nice things. I love to shop, and I love my clothes. I'm in love with fashion and I like having pretty things in my home. I enjoy going to Sephora and Bloomingdale's and seeing all the pretty things they have there. But, everytime I go on another trip, I detach a little more from my stuff. That's not to say that I don't still appreciate it, and of course I buy some souvenirs from my trips. Half the stuff in my house is stuff I've collected from the different places I've been. But, when I go to another country, I gain perspective on what really matters in life. And when I come back, I am reminded once again that my stuff doesn't own me and that I can easily live happily without it.

Here's another little anecdote, although it doesn't really have to do with traveling, more with my other point. I read "The Art of Happiness" by His Holiness the Dalai Lama on one of my trips somewhere, and I remember a part of that book that really stuck out to me. When he was talking about how much he loves going to supermarkets because he loves to look around and experience the produce section, he wrote about how much he loves to smell all the fresh produce and see all the beautiful colors, but he doesn't feel the need to buy everything or taste everything because he can still experience the joy just from being around it. I like to experience Sephora and Bloomingdales in the same way. I walk into Bloomingdales and look at all the beautiful clothes, shoes, jewelry, fragrances and everything else. The floor is beautiful, the paintings on the walls and all of the fixtures are as well. Even the way new clothes smell, I love it. But just having the experience brings me so much joy, I don't need to buy anything to have it. Of course sometimes I see something that really brings me joy and I buy it, but more often than not, I just leave with the experience. If I bought the entire store, I'd come home and not have the same joy I had while walking around. It definitely took me a few years and several thousand dollars (and trips) to realize this, but at least we're here now. We don't *need* the stuff. We have it because we like it and it brings us joy. But we know that it doesn't own us and that we can be just as happy without any of it.

PEOPLE, IN GENERAL, ARE PRETTY AMAZING AND EXTREMELY NICE, HELPFUL AND HOSPITABLE

I WENT TO TURKEY IN JANUARY of 2010. It was extremely cold. Especially for a San Diegan. I don't do well in the cold. I went to a cafe for lunch and put my jacket across my lap to keep me warm. But I was still cold. I'm always cold. I was shivering and rubbed my arms. No big deal, I wasn't freezing, but the waiter noticed this and went into a drawer and got a pashmina from it, then he came and wrapped it around my shoulders. I didn't ask for anything, he was just being kind. And it actually did help. Those pashminas are warm.

When I was in Sri Lanka with my sister in 2012, we hired a driver to take us about three hours up the coast from where we were. He didn't speak much English, and we didn't speak any Sri Lankan, so we didn't converse with him too much on the drive. Halfway through, he stopped at a fruit stand and, in his broken English and hand cues, asked us if we wanted anything, to which we said "No, thank you." I guess he just wanted to be nice and share, because he bought us a few plantains anyway, and said "Take for later," and gave them to us without asking for a dime.

When I was in Hawaii in 2011, my friend and I rented bikes. We were planning on riding bikes from our condo (about thirteen miles away) to the dock where the snorkel tour we had booked departed. About six miles in, I got a flat tire. Luckily, the rental shop had stocked us with spares, so my friend changed the tire and off we went. Five minutes later, I heard "thwop, thwop, thwop," again and looked over to see that, now, he had a flat. Once again, he changed it using the spare and off we went. Five minutes later, "thwop, thwop, thwop," again. Only this time, we didn't have another spare and it was both of our bikes. Both tires, both bikes, completely done. So we had no choice but to lock up the bikes and walk. Time was definitely of the essence, as the snorkel tour took off at a certain time and NO LATER. If we didn't get there on time, we'd lose about two hundred and fifty dollars and miss out on our all day snorkel tour! So we walked...as quickly as we could...in the rain. We kept trying to hitchhike and we even asked a couple police to take us, but they were going in the opposite direction. Finally, this guy came up to us and said "I saw y'all a little while back, but I needed to get gas because I'm going the opposite way, but I'll take you, no problem." We couldn't believe it! He drove us twenty five minutes out of his way almost halfway across part of the island to get us there, just in time. The tour was just about to pull away from the dock as we pulled up. As everyone on the boat knew about our troubles, we had about seven offers for a ride home in the first three minutes we were on the boat. And yes, we accepted a ride to the bike rental place, where (obviously) they refunded our money.

These are tiny experiences that I've had while traveling that had a big impact on me. I was in Turkey almost ten years ago and I still remember that waiter. I also had money stolen from me on a bus in Turkey, but I almost never talk about that and honestly, barely remember it. If you ask me about Turkey, the cafe story is the story I tell to show how much I loved that country. These gestures meant so much because it proved to me that people are kind. They are willing to help. They are hospitable. They are considerate. So when I come back and I see someone being rude to a server, or someone cuts me off in traffic, I remember all the good people that I've just met and the kindness I just witnessed and it makes me smile because that is what I choose to think about and what I choose to get me through the days.

THAT I'M A TEENY TINY SPECK IN THE WORLD

*T*RAVELING IS NOT THE ONLY time I've realized this (and many of the other "lessons" I've written about here) of course. I mean, all you really have to do to realize this is look up at the stars at midnight. But traveling definitely helps to put it in perspective again and again. There are billions of people in the world and you realize that when you're walking through the streets of Shanghai or watching fireworks on New Year's Eve in Brazil. It also becomes apparent when you look out the window of a plane to see the massive expanse of the Atlantic or Pacific Ocean. When I think about how much of a teeny tiny speck I am in the world, it also helps me put my "problems" in perspective. If I'm so tiny, how insignificant must the fact that my Internet isn't working right now be? So what is the point of getting worked up about it? Does it really matter in all this? Probably not. Yes, they are problems and yes, they do matter, even if it is trivial. I'm not saying that anyone should discount their own or anyone else's feelings. However, it does help to put things in perspective to see exactly which problems are worth getting worked up over. So when I feel myself getting upset about something that probably won't matter to me in a couple hours, I step back, take a breath, and ask myself whether this is something that really matters or is it something that I can most likely get past relatively easily.

NATURE IS BEAUTIFUL

I KNOW WHAT YOU'RE THINKING... "DUH! Does this lady really need to fly overseas to appreciate nature?" The answer to that question, of course, is "no." We all know nature is beautiful. I put it in here as a "lesson" because, as much as I appreciate nature in my beautiful city of San Diego, my breath has been taken away by the things I've seen in other countries. I mean, looking over cliffs in Tahiti, or swimming with whale sharks in Maldives, or staring out at the Grand Canyon, anything in the Kruger National Park in South Africa. This doesn't mean that it's any better than what I'm used to seeing. But it is different and that is the main point. Experiencing nature is always amazing. But to be able to see new scenery and animals in their natural environment is absolutely incredible. And it once again, puts everything into perspective for you, so when you return, you appreciate all the glorious nature around you. Sometimes all it takes is just a little perspective. I have a huge eucalyptus tree outside my house. My sister came to visit me for a weekend and we were sitting in my living room drinking coffee and she said "Wow, that's so awesome you have that huge tree right outside your place. If I lived here, I would just stare at it all day," and I said "I do stare at it all day." But I hadn't realized I did that until she mentioned it. But I'll sit on my couch and stare at the tree and just daydream or plan my day or whatever is on my mind. Sometimes nothing. And, I know I didn't have to travel to get this little anecdote, but she was traveling and therefore offered me a new perspective and that's part of what traveling offers-a new perspective.

THAT IF LIONS AND GAZELLES CAN COEXIST DESPITE THEIR DIFFERENCES, SO CAN BOB AND JOE FROM ACCOUNTING WHO HAVE DIFFERING POLITICAL BELIEFS

*T*HE KRUGER NATIONAL PARK IN South Africa is magical. There's really no other word to describe it. When we first drove into the park, I got chills all over my body and I almost started crying. I didn't know why and I thought I was crazy until I looked at my sister and the same thing was happening to her. Even now when we talk about it, we still both get chills and feel the same way. There are no words to explain it. It's just a feeling when the energy in the park overtakes you. We experienced some pretty amazing things while we were there as well. We fell asleep listening to (and feeling the vibrations from) lions roar. We stood about a hundred feet from a mother rhinoceros and her baby. We also saw some pretty nail biting scenes play out as well. As animal lovers, we were blown away when we saw a hyena puppy wandering around by itself. Oh my gosh, they are so freaking cute! So when it wandered over to two lions relaxing under a tree, we were almost paralyzed with fear, anticipating what we might be about to witness. Oh we were so nervous. We were holding hands, biting our lips, just waiting. This poor, sweet, adorable little puppy had know idea it just literally wandered into the lion's den. But we waited, staring, hearts pounding. The little puppy was so clueless, and it was so sweet and innocent. It didn't even turn around. The two lions laid there, staring at it, possibly contemplating what to do. This lasted for about five minutes, which probably felt like seventy five to us. Then the little pup just walked on, it crossed the road and just trotted off. The lions barely moved a muscle. They just laid there, one of them yawned, the other rolled onto her side. We couldn't believe that this little guy had just escaped death! And we were so thankful that it had! Of course we understand the animal kingdom, it's just not something we want to witness.

This wasn't the only time we witnessed this sort of thing. We saw several cheetahs at the same time that we saw a group of wildebeest parading by in a long line. There were several babies with them and many smaller ones and some older (you could tell by the way they walked). Once again, my sister and I gripped each other's hands and our hearts started pounding. We wanted to see the cheetahs run, but we didn't want to see what happened when they got to where they wanted to go. Cheetahs don't just run just to run usually. So they crept behind a couple of bushes, shoulders up and heads down, creeping like how the neighborhood cats do when we walk our dogs past. They followed each wildebeest with their eyes, and eventually the cheetahs decided for whatever reason that this was not what they wanted for dinner that night and thankfully kept walking. After seeing all this, I thought to myself, if cheetahs and wildebeest can coexist without the cheetahs killing all the wildebeest and lions just let hyena puppies and gazelles pounce past them without doing anything, why can't we? We get annoyed with a person if they chew too loudly or don't like the same shows as we do or drive too slowly. What are we thinking? My friend in high school's father used to drive so slowly and she used to always say something to him and he'd always reply "I'm driving fast enough, thank you," because to him, he was! Who are we to tell him to pick up the pace? He doesn't need to be anywhere in a hurry. Who cares? Just because someone is different than you, doesn't mean you can't live, work, and breathe next to them without letting it bother you. Just think of the lions-if they can let it (a baby hyena) go, so can you.

Now I know not all of us always have the funds and the time to travel to the Kruger or Maldives, I've been very lucky to have had the experiences I have. But, whenever and wherever you can, take these lessons. If you're on a hike, take in all the nature you possibly can. Look for signs and lessons of your own. Sometimes all you need is to look out your own window at the beautiful trees outside of your house to appreciate nature or to think of a kind gesture from one person to another that you saw at Target to remember that people are wonderful. Stay positive and keep your vibration up as much as you can and take in as much as you can from every experience. Even if all you can afford right now is camping in your backyard or a sleepover at your bestie's, do it. And fully enjoy it.

Chapter 19

ΓOLLOW THE ANIMALS

I LOVE MY DOG. I MEAN, duh, right? Everyone who has a dog loves their dog. I'm assuming you've heard someone say this once or twice, if it wasn't you. I'd venture a guess that the vast majority of pet owners would say the same thing. Sometimes, I find myself just watching her, thinking about how perfect she is and how pure and sweet and amazing she is. I know I'm not alone here. Every dog and cat (and bunny and fish) owner I know says the same thing about their pet. My dog, Naya, and I take walks everyday. We're lucky enough to live in gorgeous San Diego, so we walk along the cliffs and around the beach a lot. When I first adopted her, we frequently walked two or three hours a day because I was lucky enough to work in the evening so I had a lot of time on my hands during the day and I was able to walk for two hours a day. Even though we don't have the time to walk for three hours everyday now, our walks are still one of the most fulfilling activities that I do for so many reasons. One of the reasons I love it so much is because I try to take whatever lessons I can from her and her actions (and reactions). Animals can teach us so much if we just observe and listen to them. They are completely benevolent, innocent and loving. They also don't allow feelings and emotions to drive their actions. They don't let their past predict their future. They act from instinct and react to situations around them. When she and I are walking, to her, that's it-we're just walking, and that's all she's thinking about. One foot in front of the other. Breathe. Keep walking. Ooh look! A leaf falling! Eh, move on, keep walking, eyes front. She's not thinking about the million emails she has to write or the customer service line that she needs to call or what she's going to have for dinner.

Occasionally when we're walking, we'll walk past a fence or house that has a dog that doesn't particularly enjoy us walking past their fence, and they go a little crazy trying to get to her, fight her, bite her, play with her, maybe just tell her to get the eff away from their house, maybe trying to get to me, I'm not always sure-sometimes unclear. But, Naya is always so calm while we're walking, so she occasionally gets startled by this, and jumps a little bit, but no matter what, as soon as we're past that fence, she stops and takes a moment and just shakes it all off. She gets that good shake in to let go of whatever energy this dog has just been projecting toward her, and then she moves on. She doesn't let it affect her ever again. Ten minutes later, when we pass another dog, she doesn't bring the past into this new meeting. She is still the same, sweet dog who loves everyone. She never lets one bad experience ruin her day. To her, walking is the best activity she could ask for, it's all she ever really wants to do (well, besides run), so she just shakes it off, and moves on to enjoy the rest of the walk.

So, I try to take this lesson with me. When something happens, whether it be an angry "dog" or something else, I try to metaphorically "shake it off" and move on. Don't let other people's energy affect you or ruin your "walk" or day or drive. Shake it off and forget about it. Animals are so cool because they live in the present. They don't let yesterday or tomorrow or thirty seconds ago affect their life. If they're walking, they're walking. If they're sleeping, they're sleeping. They're not thinking about the fun they had at the dog park or the mean cat they met while out earlier that day. These are the things we can learn from them. Stay in the present. Enjoy the "now." Don't let the past dictate your future. Go into every new experience with a fresh, untainted outlook. There are so many more lessons to be taken from the animals (some of which are in the travel section of this book), these are just a few. Keep walking your dogs (and perhaps your cat or bunny or lizard if you'd like). Observe and see what you can learn from them.

Chapter 20

DO EVERYTHING WITH INTEGRITY, INTENTION AND A GOOD MOOD

*A*S I'VE SAID BEFORE, DO everything with integrity. What I haven't said is do it with a good mood. Now, I understand, we're human. To think that we're always in a good mood and that nothing ever goes wrong is absurd. So I understand it's hard to think that you can actually do EVERYTHING in a good mood. No one is always in a good mood. But, that doesn't mean that you can't still do what I'm saying. Being in a bad mood is situational and can easily be changed if you want to change it, simply from your outlook. All you have to do is switch your focus. It's that simple. If you're trying to do something and you're having trouble focusing or really getting into it because something happened before that really put you in a bad mood, stop, reset and try something else. Think, "What would my dog do?"

When I was starting my business this happened A LOT, and, y'all, I mean A LOT. If you've ever tried to start a business you know it's really freaking hard and really trying and time consuming with very little monetary payoff. So when I was starting my practice, I got really good at this. I'd sit in my office, basically just waiting for patients to walk through the door, which obviously, didn't work. People aren't just going to find you. It's not like you open your doors and people run to you screaming "Finally, an acupuncturist here! I've been looking forever!" You have to go out and find them and build your practice, just like with any business. But that's a much different topic and possibly another book. I was clearly going about it all wrong and once I switched how I was going about finding my patients, my practice finally started to pick up. However, during this time, when I was just sitting around my office, I did learn to use my time (somewhat) wisely, eventually, and even though I wasn't killing it in sales, I was still able to do some other stuff to keep progressing, at the very least. Again, since I wasn't killing it in sales, I stressed A LOT. I'd get so excited because I had a few patients scheduled and then, all of a sudden, everyone would cancel and I'd freak out, and get so stressed. I'd start questioning, "How am I going to pay my bills? How am I ever going to get this business going if I can't even get four patients?" and then immediately a patient would walk in or I'd have to talk to someone about something else. As I said, my acupuncture practice is a separate topic, but when something like this happens, and you feel like your world is crashing down and then you have to go and do something else, or talk to someone or get something done, even though you feel like your entire life is falling apart, you have to switch your focus. In this world, where we are getting text messages on our watches and emails while we're on a date, this kind of stuff happens. Not every text message is referencing happy hour at the local tavern unfortunately. I got a text message that my godfather died while I was working a Sunday afternoon shift at the bar. I got an email about my dog's (terminal) ultrasound results while I was teaching a Nutrition class. I'm sure we've all heard this at work or school or somewhere, but I know working in the restaurant industry for so long, we were often told to leave your problems at the door. This, as we know, is much easier said than done. But, we can access some good feelings even when we think we can't. Just try it.

When I say "do everything with a good mood," I also understand that sometimes it's not so easy to just switch your mood in a few seconds or breaths, although sometimes a few breaths is really all you need. So, when breathing doesn't help, do everything with integrity. You may feel discouraged sometimes and that's okay. We're human. But always do it with integrity, knowing that you're working toward your ultimate goal, whatever that may be, and that, even though you may not feel super stoked about doing it right now, the plan is still in action and it is still a step in the right direction. So you may be doing whatever you're doing saddened or upset about something else, but try to compartmentalize that as much as possible so that you don't bring those feelings into what you're trying to accomplish. It helps to think about staying present as much as possible. If you're working, focus on your work and know when you have a second to fully focus on the email you just got, you will do that. Nothing can get done all at once, and you'll never get anything done if you're half or a quarter focused on a bunch of different things. So, channel all the good feelings you can and do what you need to do now. Then, move on to the next thing with the same good feelings.

Chapter 21

FIND LOVE EVERYWHERE

*T*HERE HAVE BEEN MANY STUDIES performed showing the difference in cell structure and appearance when a person sees something he or she loves, or even hears the word "love" versus what the cell looks like when the person hears the word "hate." I even heard this same study was done on water cells (which is crazy because water isn't even alive), when someone spoke the word "love" to water versus when they said the word "hate" to water. The outcome (as I'm sure you will assume) was that the water cells appeared more beautiful and symmetrical than when exposed to "bad" feelings or hate. Now, my friends, think of what our body is mostly composed of. So, if thoughts and feelings of love can have this much effect on water, AND our body is composed mostly of water, what does that tell you? Furthermore, think about how much more complex the cells in our bodies are than water cells, so how much of an effect do you think the word "love" or even better, feelings of love have on our cells?

I know it sounds a little crazy and some of you are like "Ok, I get it. Peace, love and happiness, whatever," (eye roll), but bare with me here. Think about something or someone that you love more than anything in the world. For me, it's easy. Of course it's my dog. But it could also be the ocean and the waves or the sun and the beach. I think about how I feel when I get to the beach, when I'm about to go surfing, or when my toes hit the warm sand and when the sun hits my face. Also, when that first wave hits me and I get that salty sting on my face. It is absolutely spectacular for me, one of the best feelings ever for me. For you, it could be your cat, or your significant other, or your kids, your sister, or your parents, or a special tree in the park that you love to sit under, or the mountains, or the snow, or even a piece of art that makes you feel incredibly special. Bottom line is it could be anything. It's all about how it makes you feel. So, take a moment and think about how this thing, place, animal or person really makes you feel. Think about how much joy you get everytime you look at this thing and really feel as though you're actually there, staring at this thing, looking at it, feeling it. This is the kind of love I'm talking about. And, this feeling that you get when you see the thing we've been talking about the whole time, is so strong. It's one of the strongest feelings in the world, so strong and so powerful that it can fuel anything you want to accomplish. You may be single. You may be in a relationship. Either way, you may feel lonely at times, but you still have all the love in your heart. Feeling lonely really has nothing to do with feeling love because, no matter what, you are still surrounded by so much love, regardless of your situation, and you still have so much love in your heart to give, so why not channel it to something beneficial? So what I'm saying is, do everything with this love, channel this love when you're about to make moves and feel just as strongly as you do. Live your life with this love and this kind of power in your heart and you will be unstoppable! The first time I heard this, I was single and I angrily thought to myself "Seriously? This is ridiculous. Just because I'm single, I can't win at life? That is ridiculous!" And you know what? It *IS* ridiculous. Let me be perfectly clear: I'm not saying that AT ALL! What I'm saying is that, there is so much love in the Universe and in your heart that, no matter what your relationship status, or what you want your relationship status to be, you still are so filled with love that this is absolutely possible. So, access this love in your heart whenever, wherever you need to and do your tasks with it. Let it propel you. Let it fuel you and keep going with all the love everywhere!

Chapter 22

GET OUT THERE!

*B*ACK IN THE DAY WHEN I was contemplating quitting my bartending job and jumping fully into my acupuncture practice, a wise woman said to me "Sarah, no one ever gets off a comfy couch, so get off the couch on YOUR terms." The Universe, or God, or whatever you believe in has a way of making things you want to happen, happen. However, if you wait around to let it happen, it might not happen in the way you want it to. If you're thinking about quitting your job to go into another career path, you may get a horrible new boss, or (geez, hopefully not) maybe the place you work closes or gets shut down for some reason. If something like this happens, you're left scrambling and making quick fast decisions to make your next move. You're not able to really think about, prepare and get yourself ready to do what it is you're planning to do. So, make whatever you want to happen, happen-in the way you want it to. And the way you make it happen in the way you want it to is by getting off the couch, getting out there and doing it your damn self. I mean honestly, can you think of a better way? No one is going to make you do anything and they are also not going to do it for you.

Years and years ago, when I first moved to San Diego, I went into outside sales for a very short time. I was twenty five and had no idea what outside sales even meant, so I thought to myself, hey, I get to be outside, right? That's cool! That's why I moved to San Diego in the first place! So why not? So I tried it. And I HATED it. I mean, I really did not like it at all. Sales is a fantastic career and there is a great amount of money to be made doing it, just not by me. I just really did not enjoy cold calling and going into businesses, without an appointment, trying to talk to someone and sell them something. I was always so uncomfortable. I've come to enjoy sales way more than I used to, but this particular job was just not for me. So I lasted a few months doing outside sales, but I quickly put the wheels in motion to find a bartending job so that I didn't do that very long. I ended up bartending much longer than I had anticipated or even meant to and after several years of working in the bar industry and attending Chinese Medical school and getting my doctorate, I started my acupuncture practice. After I was in practice for a while, I started my own skincare line. With these two ventures, guess what I found myself doing...going into (and calling and following up with) stores and shops and salons and day spas and doctors' offices and all kinds of places that I was not comfortable calling on. It reminded me so much of my very brief stint doing outside sales. I'd get so nervous and uncomfortable and start sweating in such weird places and I'd walk into these places and just think I must look like the biggest idiot on the face of the earth, why in the hell would anyone want to refer patients to me or sell my skincare? I can barely even pronounce skincare! I'd fall all over my words, start stuttering, and pretty much revert back to my six year old self, who was so shy, my voice cracked by just saying hi. So, each time I'd do this, I'd give myself a little pep talk before I walked in. I'd listen to gangster rap in my car on the way to each new business. I'd channel all the love I had in my heart and think how much I loved helping people and that this is going to help me reach more people so I can help them. So I did it. I did it one time. Then I did it twice, and then three times, and every time I did it, it got easier and easier. My script got better, to the point that I had perfected it after just a few trips. What else I found was, ninety nine times out of a hundred, people were extremely nice. They were always so interested in what I was doing and what my mission was. I know, I know, Acupuncture and Chinese herb and crystal infused skincare does sound a little more intriguing than when I was selling phone systems and some other stuff that people are out there selling. But, even if they wanted nothing to do with my product or services (which definitely happened plenty of times too, believe me!), they were still so nice and cordial in telling me "Not right now." So basically, every time I did it, it just got easier and easier to walk through that door or pick up the phone and I promise you it will be the same for you, regardless of what you're out there doing!

The first time is always the hardest, no matter what you're doing. No matter what you're doing, you most likely won't be a pro at it immediately. I've taught many people how to do a cartwheel and the first thing I always say to them is "No one came out of their mother cartwheeling, right?" It may take a little while, it may be a little uncomfortable, you may not do it perfectly immediately, but you just have to take the plunge, do it one time and after that, it's all downhill, so just keep at it. It's all about perseverance. Keep trying. Keep doing it. Keep at it. It'll keep getting easier and easier every time and eventually, there you go! Furthermore, as anyone in sales will tell you, it's all a numbers game. If you go into a hundred doors, ninety nine might say no, but you're focused on that one yes. And every "no" is another chance to learn and it's another tick in the box that is getting you closer to the "yes." This is not new knowledge. We just have to access it sometimes.

No matter what you're trying to do or accomplish, you must get out there. Sometimes you have to get up from a comfortable couch, figuratively or literally. Sometimes it's all about repetition and just getting those reps in makes it easier and easier. If you want to run a marathon, you have to get off the couch and train. You're not just going to run 26.2 miles if you've been sitting on the couch for the past three months. Get those reps in. Get off the couch! Run a mile the first time, run two the next. It'll keep getting easier and easier, but if you never start, you'll never get anywhere.

If you're trying to make a big move in your career, get off the couch. Do some research. Get out there. Go on some interviews, see who's hiring, see what you need to do and what moves you need to make (and then make them!) to get where you want to be! In the words of Nike, "Just do it!"

Chapter 23

ALLOWANCE

*R*EMEMBER WHEN YOU WERE A kid and your parents used to give you an allowance? Growing up, I always thought that was the only definition of that word. What else could it mean, except the money your parents give you on Saturday so that you can go buy some gum and fruity smelling chapstick? It wasn't until I was an adult doing all my mindset manifestation work on myself that I realized allowance had a slightly different meaning. Allowance, according to mirriam-webster.com, means (among other definitions) "the act of allowing something." How simple is that definition? It's so great, right? How easy is that? All you have to do is *ALLOW* things into your life. You don't need to wrangle and fight and wrestle all these things into your world. *ALLOW* yourself to make more money and have a wonderful job. *ALLOW* yourself to have the beautiful body outside that reflects who you know you are inside. *ALLOW* the love of your life to come to you. Now, this is all fine and great, right? Sounds so easy and you're all like "Hello! What do you think I've been doing for the last five years! Duh, of course I'm *allowing* myself these things." But are you, really? Really look into yourself. Are you really *allowing*? Or is it possible that you are resisting? You may not even realize that you are, in fact, resisting. But, it's this resistance that is pushing things away from yourself. And, what I mean by you could possibly be resisting, when you think you're allowing is, this. When you go to the bathroom and look at yourself in the mirror and think "Ugh, I look terrible. I haven't even lost a pound," you are resisting your beautiful body. When you think to yourself "I would rather pull my own teeth out than go meet this online date for coffee," (which I have definitely said, btw) you are resisting the love of your life entering your world. When you wake up in the morning and think "if I make it through this day at work, it'll be a miracle," that's resisting that amazing new job. When you're resisting what you want to come into your life, essentially you're pushing it away from you. What is wonderful, is that it is so easy to switch it from resistance to allowance. All you have to do is switch the focus. Instead of saying "Ugh I look terrible, I haven't lost a pound," say "I am on the right track. I am doing everything I can and I know I am making progress. I allow my body to be the beautiful physicality that I know it is and that reflects who I am on the inside." Instead of saying "I would rather pull out my own teeth, than meet this person for coffee," say "Even if this doesn't turn out to be my person, I may have a wonderful conversation and I am one step closer to getting to my person. I know they are out there and I allow them to enter my life." All you have to do is switch the focus, just switch the script. And honestly, it really is that easy, although it does take practice and time to really understand it and not have to consciously tell yourself to switch the focus. Nothing really happens overnight, so it will take practice for you before you start walking into every Bumble date with a positive, happy outlook, regardless of the outcome, or not getting discouraged when you step on the scale and have gained two pounds even though you've worked out every day and eaten nothing but broccoli and tuna all week. I get it, it's hard to keep that "allowance attitude." It's very easy to get discouraged when it seems like there are no jobs, no love prospects, no pounds lost, etc. but honestly, won't it feel better to have a positive happy outlook regardless? Do you really enjoy feeling bad? I know you don't, or you wouldn't be reading this book. So even if it doesn't happen overnight, doesn't it still feel better to not hate your body, or not have a terrible attitude with every first date when it comes to finding the love of your life? It will happen, and in the meantime, you can start feeling better anyway. Seems like a win win, right?

Chapter 24

RELINQUISH CONTROL

*W*HEN MY FIANCE AND I got engaged, we were ecstatic. Duh, right? We were so happy. I couldn't believe how happy and in love I was. The entire year of our engagement felt like that. Every time we accomplished something else or checked something off the wedding to do list, we got happier and happier and more and more excited. We got engaged in April and by Christmas that year I remember going to bed every night thinking "I'm so happy this is my life." Everything was going great and I was so happy and so excited for what the next day held. Then January came. My beloved dog, Naya (who I've written about extensively in this book), started losing weight. She had always been skinny, but she started looking really skinny. At first we thought it was because I wasn't walking or running with her anymore. She had arthritis and when I'd try to walk her, she'd get sore and limp for a day or two after, so I stopped. So we didn't think it was that big of a deal at first. She seemed so healthy, but we wanted to take her to the vet anyway, just to be sure everything was alright. They took blood and saw that one of her liver enzymes was elevated, so they ordered an ultrasound, which revealed several tumors on her liver, spleen and ribs. It was only shortly after that (about a week) that she died. It was the end of January that we had to say goodbye. We were devastated. She was my best friend and for a long time, my only family in San Diego. We had just met with our wedding coordinator earlier that week and we discussed what the dogs would be doing during the ceremony and reception and I had just asked one of my friends to be in charge of them during the ceremony. I was planning what each of the dogs was going to wear, where they would sleep, who would be in charge of keeping the gates locked and everything else. It happened so quickly it just seemed like she got yanked out of my arms and into the sky and now she was gone. I was extremely sad for a long time, and honestly, I'll never stop missing her. But after a couple months or so, I started smiling again, I started laughing and I started looking forward to the wedding again. It was so hard to even try to get excited about anything for so long after she died, but then finally I accepted the fact that she was gone and not going to be at the wedding, but we knew it would still be great. So we started planning again. I was ordering all the last minute small detailed things, like lanterns and lights and really started to get excited all over again. It was right around early March of 2020 that our house was filled with boxes of ribbons and crystals and all kinds of decor. Most of you reading, I'm sure, remember March of 2020. It was when we really started to get worried about CoronaVirus. It was about then that people from out of town started texting me to say they weren't sure they'd be able to make it. Then we started seeing news articles saying big events, concerts, shows, were getting canceled and rescheduled. We really started getting worried when the government issued cancellations of any event over two hundred fifty people, but still thought maybe there was a chance. Our wedding wasn't going to be that big, maybe we'd be fine, right? Hopefully??? But as the days (well, hours) went on, it just kept getting worse and worse, and finally a few days later, we decided we had no choice but to postpone the wedding. Once again, we were devastated. It seemed like the Universe was messing with me. I kept thinking what the actual fuck? Is this really happening? Like, what the hell? And that was my mentality for a little while again, I'll be honest. I did not handle it as well as I'd like to tell most people. I felt like a victim, like all this was being done to me. I mean, first my dog, then our wedding. But, once again, after I accepted that this was what was actually happening and it wasn't some terrible dream, I took a step back and just simply came to the realization that I have no control over anything. It's pretty hard for a lot of us to relinquish control, but once we realize that we don't really have control over anything anyway, we need to just let it happen as it's going to happen. Now, this is not to say that you shouldn't work towards goals or do your manifestations and vision boards (believe me, I've been there). I had the "Why try?" mentality for a little while when all this was happening, because again, I felt like a victim. I felt like, if everything was just going to happen the way it was going to happen anyway, why the heck should I try and work so hard to do what I'm trying to do when the Universe is just going to decide to do whatever it wants to do anyway? And, I can't sit here and tell you the answer to that question, because I still really don't totally know the answer. Yes, I know from experience that manifesting and working toward goals works. However, if we could manifest our pets to live forever, *of course*, we'd all have thirty seven year old dogs running alongside us, right? So, obviously, it doesn't work like that. We're all still mortal and life still happens. What I do know is that you have to relinquish control. As hard as it is to say and do, you just have to realize that you don't really have control over a lot of things anyway. What you do have control over, is your response to it; your emotions, your perspective and your reactions. I could've decided to suffer, to let my pain take over when Naya died and then to let my sadness take over when our wedding got postponed. I could've thought "Why is this happening to me?" Honestly, I did for a little while. But, much like we all do through life, we put on our leggings, throw our hair in a bun, and deal with it. Why? Because as we know, a bun is the best way to look put together when everything seems to be falling apart. We also know, at the end of the day, no one is doing this *to you*. The Universe doesn't have it out for you, it's not fucking with you. Sometimes life happens and, as I said, we don't have control over it, so we can choose to react in a way that is beneficial and constructive for us and move forward with what we're given and learn from our experiences. Or we can choose to react in a way that is destructive for us and with a victim mentality that doesn't really help anything at all. But again, the choice is yours. What would you choose? To live in misery, or build yourself back up? Seems simple when you're not going through it, but believe me, it's not as easy when you're living it. So, if you find yourself wrapped up in your pain, letting yourself suffer, remember, sure it could be better, but it could always be worse. Remember some things you're grateful for, think about some things that bring you joy. And be thankful for the memories that you do have. When I think about Naya now, when I think about the day we got engaged, it brings me so much joy and I'm so grateful she was there for that and with me for as long as she was. I have wonderful memories of her for the twelve years that she and I were together that I will always remember and I know our wedding will be great whenever it happens. Remember the things that made you happy in the first place and be grateful for them, and then, start planning your next move. Where do we go from here? What do you need to do to make yourself feel happy, get back on track and get stuff done? Let's do those things!

Chapter 25

KINDNESS AND LIVING CLEAN

WHEN I SAY "LIVING CLEAN" I don't totally mean you can't ever use styrofoam (although I know we all despise it and it would be great if you could totally eliminate it from your life, but it's just not reasonable to think you'll completely eliminate it from your life forever. Eventually it's going to creep back in at some point, unfortunately. But, we can try to use it sparingly by bringing reusable containers when we go out to eat and bringing our own water bottles places and stuff like that and try to reduce our consumption of it and other disposable containers as much as we can. But I digress..) or that you have to give up your French fries with ranch dressing or Aperol spritzes forever. We're human and you have to allow yourself to be human now and then. Should you try to remember to pack a reusable container in your purse for your leftovers when you go out to eat? Of course! Are you going to forget it once in a while and have to ask for a box? Yep, you are. Will you be on a road trip and have to buy a plastic bottle of iced tea from the gas station, or go to a different country and end up with a styrofoam container of noodles or rice? Duh! You're human! Are you going to eat french fries and want to dip them in ranch every now and then? Who doesn't? It's freaking delicious! These are things that we all do (some of which we love, even though they're not the healthiest or the most carbon neutral choice we've ever made). But, as I've said, we're human and we make mistakes and we travel and sometimes live for convenience. So, this is not necessarily what I'm talking about when I say "living clean."

What I mean when I say "living clean" is to get rid of the excess "clutter" in your life. We all watched Marie Kondo, right? Get that crap outta here! Not just in your condo, but in all aspects. If it doesn't bring you joy, or move you forward in some way, be done with it. Maybe your job doesn't really bring you joy. But, maybe it's a stepping stone to where you want to be or where you need to go. Get rid of it? Maybe not yet. Buuuuuuttttt, maybe you can start looking in another direction to get yourself where you do want to be. So when I say live clean and Marie Kondo your life, I mean evaluate every decision you make, whether it's "Do I want to eat this deep dish pizza?" Or "Should I quit my job?" Or "Should I move to another state?" And, even "Do I want to continue talking to this person?" Yes, I'm talking about toxic relationships as well!

So yes, living clean can mean eating clean, getting rid of clutter, reducing your carbon footprint, all of it. But it can also mean getting rid of the crap that doesn't bring you joy and moving toward the things that do. So from now on, when it comes to your decision making process, think to yourself, does it bring me joy or fulfill me in some sort of way? If it does not, it's a no. If there's any part of you that says "Maybe I don't want to do this," reevaluate it! If you're trying to move in a different direction with your job or get a whole other job completely and you get an offer to stay in the same basically stagnant or do a lateral move, do you want to take it? Possibly, but do an evaluation to see if it is an absolute yes, if it's not, it's a no. I'm also a huge fan of pros and cons lists! Anything you're unsure of, make a pro and con list. Look at the list and then see how you feel. For example, if it's a job and you make a pro and con list with all the pros and cons of staying in your current job and another of all the pros and cons of leaving. First, (obviously) see which list wins, and then see how you feel when you look at the winning list. Is it what you were hoping? Is it what you truly feel inside yourself is the best decision for yourself and your future? If it's not, stop! Reevaluate, meditate, think what would truly, truly bring you joy and make a plan as to how to make that happen! If it doesn't bring you joy, it's out! If it's not a whole hearted yes, it's a no!

Continue to do this with every decision you make in every aspect of your life. Are you working towards the body you've always wanted? The physical being that you know you are inside that just hasn't been reflected on the outside, and you're working hard toward this. Everyday you do an awesome workout, and you're logging your food in some calorie counting app or something like that, eating clean, knowing what you're putting into your body is exactly right, in the exact right portions. But then one day, one of your friends says they've been craving nachos and margaritas and were hoping you'd join them. Once you get to the restaurant, evaluate your choices-you could have five margaritas, a burrito, some chips and salsa, and go ahead and add guacamole, and sure, some sour cream too! You could have none of that, order a sparkling water with a lemon and a side salad with the dressing you brought from home and pour water on the chips when they come to the table so you don't eat any of them. Your friend wouldn't be too happy with you if you did that, I'm sure. Or, you could order a skinny margarita, have a few chips and salsa and indulge in a couple tacos with grilled fish or chicken. Which of these options seems like the best choice to you? I mean, it seems obvious, but really, it's whichever option would be an absolute yes to you. Are you going to feel fulfilled ordering a sparkling water and saying no to chips and salsa? Maybe, but maybe you might feel like you're depriving yourself. Are you going to feel fulfilled ordering five margs, a burrito and guacamole? Maybe for a while, but I guarantee, if you've been eating clean for several months and you eat all this food, you will feel sick later on and most likely unfulfilled. But, if you're still willing to risk it and it seems like an absolute yes to you, go for it! But I honestly don't think it would be an absolute yes for you. I think we can all agree that indulging a little and not going overboard will probably feel best and you won't worry about it derailing all your efforts until now.

So once again, start applying living clean in ALL aspects of your life, find the choice that's going to bring you the most joy. Declutter your life, get the stuff (people, tv shows, activities, jobs, whatever) out that doesn't bring you joy and if it's not a total and complete yes, it's a no and move on.

Chapter 26

WHEN EVERYTHING SUCKS

*I*T TOOK ME A WHILE to write this book, almost two years (some would say way longer than it should have). While writing, unfortunately, as I've said, my sweet dog, Naya, passed away. It was one of the worst things I've had to go through ever and basically, it sucked. Everything sucked for a while. I felt like I was high all the time and none of the time because I was totally out of it but never happy. I felt like I was floating, but not in a good way. I didn't know how to get through the day and all I wanted to do was lie in bed or on the couch and watch murder stories. I thought the pain would never go away and I just cried and cried and cried and then cried more. I was angry with the Universe for taking my baby away from me so quickly. It felt like she was just yanked out of my hands and gone forever. I cried and complained and wondered why the hell this was happening? I felt like it was so unfair and in some way, (selfishly) I felt like it was happening *TO* me and I couldn't understand why. I had written in my gratitude journal every day, and every day I was grateful for her; for all the memories we have together, for all the runs, for the fact that she was here now and so was I. Each day I wrote something else about her and our life. I love her so much and I couldn't imagine a day without her. I didn't want to. Maybe I thought if I kept writing how grateful I was for her being here, it would somehow keep her here, which, in a way, really is trying to cheat and we all know that's not gonna work. And at the very end, we knew we didn't have a lot of time, so my super sweet sister got us a session with a professional pet photographer. On Tuesday, I booked a session with her for Saturday. Naya died Wednesday. She didn't even make it until the weekend, so I had to cancel the appointment. I had been so excited to get these photos and I was so angry with the Universe that it couldn't even give me that. I just wanted some nice photos at her favorite spot (Sunset Cliffs) to have and frame and the Universe couldn't even give me that. I was so angry. I kept looking into it, trying to find the lesson. Why couldn't she have hung on just a little longer? Why couldn't we at least have the photos? I didn't know. I still don't know. But it's also not for me to know and, really, it doesn't matter. It wasn't about me and I had to realize that. It was about Naya and the Universe and for whatever reason, they both had decided that it was Naya's time to go and I just had to accept that; not the easiest thing I've had to do. Have I by now? Wellllllllllllllllll, it's still a work in progress, but I'm getting there. I have accepted it, but, of course, still miss her everyday.

As you have read, Naya and I were always runners. She is, still to this day, the best running partner I've ever had, so that was the only thing I could do to get myself to move. It made me feel so close to her again, so, much like Forrest Gump, I ran. As hard as it was to get out of bed, I made myself do it for her. To feel her presence while I was running made me so happy and so sad all at once, but I just let myself cry, because hey, I was by myself and already sweating, so who would know or care? Did running help? For the most part, yes. But honestly, nothing *REALLY* helped. The bottom line is sometimes things just plain suck. When your dog dies, that sucks and there isn't anything you or anyone else can do or say that is going to make that not suck. I didn't write in my gratitude journal for three weeks straight. Sure, there were things to be grateful for, there are always things to be grateful for and I knew that, but I just didn't feel like writing in it. Is it the best thing to do? Maybe not, but I was sad, and I didn't feel like looking for things to make me happy or make my life better. When things suck like that, sometimes you just have to let them suck, you're human, and that's okay. But, the lesson is to not let yourself fall into the suckiness for too long. Yes, I neglected my gratitude journal for a couple weeks, but I went outside and ran, I breathed, I meditated and let Naya's light shine on me while I did. I showered and I put my hair in a bun and I went to the office and treated patients. I taught my Spin classes and I taught my Nutrition classes. I did what I had to do, but with a fuzzy layer over everything. Sometimes you just have to put your hair in a bun, put on some leggings and go through the motions, as I've said. Let yourself mourn, give yourself a break, get angry, feel it, get sad, feel it more, but don't let it engulf you. Keep moving, so that you don't fall into the suck. If you let yourself fall into the suck (or get "sucked" in...see what I did there?), you're in danger of letting it become you. Things are going to go bad. You're going to experience loss, tragedy, sadness and pain. But if you let yourself fall into that sadness or pain, that becomes you and that's not you! You can let yourself experience the sadness, pain and tragedy, but just don't let it become you. Know that it won't last and take steps to make sure it doesn't last. Let it suck, but just don't let it suck too long.

Chapter 27

BE PATIENT

*W*E'RE ALWAYS LOOKING FORWARD TO the next thing, right? I can't wait until my vacation. I can't wait til Friday. I can't wait til Christmas! We're all guilty of this and that's okay. Patience is a funny thing. Some of us are very patient, some (myself included) are not. Some of us (actually, this is more myself) are patient for some things, but for other things, you better watch out. You can ask a lot of people that know me. I'm not very patient at all. Well, with some things I am, some not so much. I'm pretty patient with people in my clinic, and the people around me, not so patient with people driving in front of me. I try to be patient, I even have a tattoo on my arm reminding me to be patient. It doesn't help. When I focus on something, I want it NOW. I mean RIGHT NOW. When I started school, I just wanted to graduate. When I got engaged, I just wanted my wedding day to come! What I've had to learn is that the Universe doesn't really work that way. I can be on one timeline, yet the Universe is clearly on another. I have been reminded of this over and over and over again, but finally when my wedding had to be postponed because of CoronaVirus, I was sure the Universe and I were on different timelines.

But still, if I want to lose 50lbs. I want it gone tomorrow. If I want to buy a house, I want to start packing, tonight. This drives my fiance crazy. He tells me all the time to just relax. Like I said, when I focus on something, that's it. Nothing will stop me until I get it. Now, this isn't necessarily a bad thing. It's great to keep focused on goals and things you want to accomplish. Otherwise, what are we doing? Why do we have vision boards and goal sheets and things like that? I'm saying that, as you're working toward your goals, just understand that it may not happen in the time that you're hoping and just know that that's okay because it *will* happen. As long as you keep working toward it, and moving forward, and manifesting/praying/projecting energy (whatever you do), it *will* happen. Don't let the "not on your timeline" discourage you. Just know that it might not happen tomorrow, but the joy of learning from it will also be fun. The journey and failures are how we learn and that is what will teach you the lessons.

The other thing, though, is I'm not saying say "F it," and "let the Universe figure it out," and just stop working toward it, or put everything off until tomorrow either. There is a balance between these two ideas. Basically what I'm saying is yes, by all means, focus on your goals, make your vision boards, do all the moon manifestations and prayers and tarot cards and everything else you want to manifest the amazing life that you want, but be happy with where you are along the way. Look at each place in your journey and get excited about the "now" and know that what you are working toward is happening, but also, let it go if it doesn't happen on *your* timeline. The plan is fluid and you may think you're ready for something but a higher intelligence may know you're not. You may want to make partner or get a certain promotion by the time you're *this* age. Maybe you want to lose *this* many pounds by *this* date. Maybe you want to get married by the time you're *this* age. The Universe may have another timeline and a purpose for it, so understand that and simply accept it, but don't give up. As I said, this is one of the lessons I've had to work on A LOT in my life. When I want something, I want it NOW, so I understand this. But this is also why I now understand patience and giving it up to the Universe and knowing that there is a higher power that knows more than I do, and therefore, has a reason for not giving it to me now. One of those reasons, I believe, is for the emotions you get to experience along the journey. Think about when you are losing weight. Have you ever watched a weight loss show on TV? I have, many times. I've spent a lot of time in gyms over the years and I've seen and heard many amazing, inspiring weight loss journeys. Now just imagine this is you. You get on the scale one morning and make the firm decision you are going to change your life by finally losing the weight you've been talking about losing for years. This is the day. You even snap a couple "before" photos on your phone as your starting point. You put on some sneakers and a pair of shorts and walk out the door. You try to run a little, but it's pretty hard, it's been years since you've gone for an actual run. So mostly you walk, but you work up a pretty good sweat. This is actually way harder than you thought. "Am I really this out of shape?" you think to yourself. You come home, you shower and you look in your fridge to find not too much, so you make the healthiest option there, which is eggs for breakfast. So, you make a plan to go to the supermarket later. You buy all the healthy things-tons of veggies, fish, chicken, some fruit, and a couple of healthy carbs (high fiber, sprouted, whatever). And now you're feeling pretty good. This is it! You're going to actually do this! You make a delicious, healthy dinner and go to sleep feeling great. The next morning, you wake up, you're pretty sore from your exercise yesterday, but what do you do? You put on your sneakers and walk out the door again. This time, you push yourself a little harder, run a little further, even though you're sore and come home and make yourself a delicious, healthy, breakfast. Throughout the day, your soreness gets worse. You have to hold yourself up when you walk up and down your stairs, everything aches, but in a good way. You know you worked and you still feel great. You make another delicious healthy dinner that night, and again, go to sleep feeling great. You keep this up for a week and finally get on the scale to find you've lost four pounds! All this hard work has started to pay off and you are on your way! It gives you great motivation to keep going and you look back on the week and think "I did great! That was all me and my own motivation! Go me!" This continues for several weeks, and you start going back to the gym and finally start using that membership you've been paying for every month, but never using. You start following fitness and health pages on social media, and start experimenting with your meals, always keeping it healthy. Your friends and coworkers start making comments to you, not only, about how great you look, but how happy you seem and how much more you're smiling lately. From then, this just continues and keeps getting better. You keep checking the scale each week and you keep losing. Your pants are getting looser and you have to buy new clothes, and when you go shopping, you feel so happy. Everything looks amazing on you and it just keeps getting better and better until you finally hit your goal! You made it! You feel so amazing and accomplished and proud of yourself! All your hard work, dedication, discipline and effort has paid off! You look in the mirror and you are so happy to see the person looking back at you. The journey was tough, but it was so worth it and now you are here, feeling great, looking great! It is amazing how wonderful you feel!

Now just imagine you got on the scale one morning, once again, told yourself you were going to lose weight and did nothing about it. That day you woke up, showered, had some coffee and then a couple donuts at the office. You sat at your desk watching Facebook videos for the majority of the day and then went home, opened a bottle of wine and ate chips and salsa for dinner. The next morning you woke up and, as if you were in some Tom Hanks movie, you looked in the mirror and then got on the scale and you were miraculously at your goal weight. Without even trying or doing anything at all, you dropped fifteen (or however many) pounds! Yes, it sounds like this would be the better option and that it would be so easy, why can't this actually happen? Of course, you want something for doing nothing, it's like winning the lottery! But think, if it did, you would have been robbed all these months of working toward your goal and getting to feel the emotions of winning and hitting tiny goals. Every time you go shopping, or you put on clothes, you feel better and better and these feelings get stronger and stronger as you keep working toward the main goal. These feelings wouldn't feel as good, if you didn't do the work and get to feel all of them as you're working and the good emotions compound on each other, so you just keep feeling happier and happier through your journey. I promise. I know you're thinking, "No, I'd be pretty happy if I won the lottery or if I woke up and had the body I've always wanted." You're right, you would be. But you wouldn't have the same sense of satisfaction, accomplishment and gratification that you'll get from doing the work and manifesting it on your own. Of course there will be ups and downs, as there always is, when you're working toward something. But again, it just makes it all worth it in the end, and I promise, the ultimate feeling is so much better than it would've been, had it happened exactly how you planned in the exact perfect timing or with zero effort whatsoever. This story is actually a story from one of my lovely patients. She came to see me the whole time and I saw her progress and her transition. Her goal was to lose thirty pounds and she was hoping to do it in six months. It ended up taking her almost a year to hit her goal weight, but throughout her weight loss journey, she just kept up, and I witnessed her growing and becoming more confident and happy throughout the entire time. Witnessing her transition really helped to solidify the theory that the journey is what makes it all worth it. I loved seeing her attitude change, and I know she loved seeing herself change.

SOME FINAL WORDS

$\mathcal{O}$K, SO I KNOW I'VE thrown a lot at you over the last hundred or so pages, but these are all ideas to help you live your best life. Take a few that really stand out to you and start practicing those. As you get used to doing those few, add a few more in and see how you feel. Keep going with anything that resonates with you and keep feeling better and better. See how your life or your attitude changes (most likely both) as you start feeling better. However, always keep in mind that this, just like anything else is a "practice" and requires practice like any sport or activity you've ever picked up. Don't lose faith or get discouraged when you have a bad day and always be patient and gentle with yourself. As I always say, talk to yourself as you would talk to your best friend. Don't beat yourself up for missing a couple days or getting bummed every once in a while. You are a human and you will have bad days and you will feel like being lazy every now and then. Sometimes "self care" means sitting around the house watching home renovation shows or reality TV all day, whatever you need on that day is fine. Always just be sure to keep moving on and allow yourself the time you need to do what you need to do, but get back to the practice (whichever ones they may be) after that. Remember, don't let yourself fall into the "suck." Always make sure you're moving forward and just don't give up! You'll get there, even if it takes you a million years (which, I promise, it won't if you keep going).

I'm also here to tell you it won't be perfect. Life won't be perfect. The process won't be perfect. Your plan may seem perfect, but I promise you the plan will change and other stuff will come up that won't be so perfect. Basically, you just have to get the word "perfection" out of your head. Stop trying to make yourself perfect. You're human, you're beautifully imperfect and you will make mistakes. Therefore, the things you do and the plans you make will also be beautifully imperfect. The less perfect you try to be, the easier your life will be, seriously. Trust me, life gets a lot easier when you stop trying to make it perfect. If you just try as hard as you can to be the best version of yourself that you can be, you will be a lot happier and you will get a lot more accomplished, I promise!

The things I've said in this book are all ideas to help you continue moving forward in life. We don't want to become complacent or stagnant, so it's always helpful to have a few extra ideas in place for when you start feeling that way. As I said before, start small and keep adding things into your repertoire. Keep this book somewhere that is easily accessible, so when you're feeling stagnant you can just refer back to it and find something new to try. And, when you've tried it all, go back again and redo some stuff. Always make sure you're moving forward, working toward something, making yourself better and making yourself *feel* better. Sometimes we don't know how good we can feel until we realize we feel better than we did before, so if you think you're already at one hundred, just keep up with what you're already doing and see if you can add something else into the mix to see if you can get your vibration a little higher! And while you're doing all this keep congratulating yourself and acknowledging all of your achievements thus far! The idea is to continue feeling good, not to start making yourself feel bad. Know that you're awesome exactly how you are! And you can be even more awesome by keeping up with all the fun tools that we've talked about, but don't ever talk yourself out of knowing that (and feeling like) you are the coolest person you know. The minute you stop feeling like you're a total badass is the minute you'll stop wanting to work on yourself and you'll really want to give up. Always remember you look, feel and do things great all the time and if you continue working on yourself, you'll be, feel, look and do things even more great! As I've stressed and stressed so much throughout this book, I know it's not reasonable to think that you actually will feel (or look) great *all* the time, but just make sure you don't let yourself fall into the suckiness. Let yourself feel the feelings that you want to feel, and then let them go and move on. Get back on track and continue getting your life together! The reason I do what I do is because

I enjoy helping people feel better and It has been my pleasure writing this book, imagining helping all of you get healthier and feel better! I really hope some of these ideas have stuck out to you and you will use some of them in your life, and if you need any help at all, let me know! I'll be over here, taking a nap (just kidding)!